Get a Good Night's Sleep

Understand Your Sleeplessness— and Banish it Forever!

Frank J. Bruno, Ph.D.

Macmillan • USA

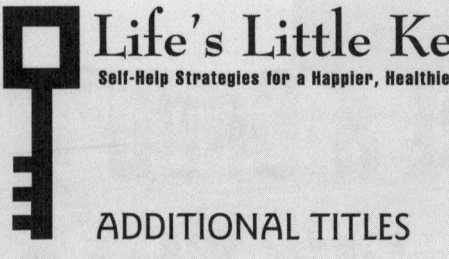

Life's Little Keys
Self-Help Strategies for a Happier, Healthier You

ADDITIONAL TITLES

Stop Worrying

Conquer Shyness

Stop Procrastinating

Defeat Depression

Conquer Loneliness

*To those who struggle
with the problem of insomnia*

Copyright © 1997 by Frank Bruno
All rights reserved including the right of reproduction
in whole or in part in any form.

Macmillan General Reference
A Simon & Schuster Macmillan Company
1633 Broadway
New York, NY 10019-6785

An Arco Book

MACMILLAN is a registered trademark
of Macmillan, Inc.
ARCO is a registered trademark of Prentice-Hall, Inc.

ISBN: 0-02-861306-6
Library of Congress Catalog Card Number: 96-085341

Manufactured in the United States of America
10 9 8 7 6 5 4 3 2 1

Cover design by Kevin Hanek
Book design by Scott Meola

CONTENTS

    Preface   vii
    Acknowledgments   viii

1 *Kinds of Sleep Difficulties:*
    "I Couldn't Sleep a Wink Last Night"   1

2 *Understanding a Normal Sleep Pattern:*
    From Deep Sleep to Light Sleep
    and Back Again   13

3 *Emotions and Sleep:*
    Blues in the Night   29

4 *The Meaning of Dreams:*
    The Need for REM Sleep   45

5 *When Life Is Disorganized:*
    Forming Good Sleep Habits   65

6 *Self-Hypnosis:*
    A Practical Sleep-Induction Skill   81

7 *More Ways to Obtain Better Sleep:*
    A Catalog of Tips and Techniques   93

8 *Professional Assistance:*
    Medical Treatments and Psychotherapy   115

9 *A Seven-Step Anti-Insomnia Program*   131

PREFACE

It's 2:00 A.M.

You've been trying to fall asleep since 11:00 P.M. Three miserable hours have passed. You're not sick. As far as you know, you don't have an illness that is causing you to be wide awake when you don't want to be.

What do you do?

Do you just suffer?

Do you take a sleeping pill?

Is there a better way to cope with the problem of insomnia than to play the role of victim?

There *is* a better way, and this book directs you toward it. Or, perhaps, the reference should be to better *ways*. There is no single royal road to the land of dreams. Instead, there are various coping strategies that are likely to be effective, depending on individual differences between people.

The numerous self-directed coping strategies in *Get a Good Night's Sleep* are presented as a set of tips and techniques. These will, if applied with will and positive attitude, enable you to obtain health-giving rest.

ACKNOWLEDGMENTS

A number of people have helped me make *Get a Good Night's Sleep* a reality. My thanks are expressed to:

Barbara Gilson, senior editor at Macmillan, for her recognition of the value of the book and for being a supportive and creative editor.

Jennifer Perillo, editor at Macmillan, for her assistance and for her appreciation of the book's themes.

George J. McKeon, artist, for his capturing of key ideas in cartoon form.

Bert Holtje, my agent, for encouraging the development of the book.

Diane Pfahler, a colleague and psychology instructor, for making some useful observations about personality traits and sleep.

Ron Ruiz, a colleague and psychology instructor, for pointing out how the hum of a fan can sometimes be useful for inducing sleep.

George K. Zaharoupoulos, an exceptional colleague, for his steadfast encouragement of my writing projects.

My wife, Jeanne, for our many meaningful discussions.

My son, Franklin, for our conversations about language and meaning.

1 KINDS OF SLEEP DIFFICULTIES: "I COULDN'T SLEEP A WINK LAST NIGHT"

Do you find it difficult to fall asleep when you go to bed?

Do you wake up in the middle of the night, and then find it hard to go back to sleep?

Do you wake up much earlier in the morning than you want to?

Do you do a lot of tossing and turning most nights?

Do you feel drowsy or sluggish during the day because you are sleep deprived?

In brief, is the general quality of your life diminished because you can't get a good night's sleep?

If you answered one or several questions with a *yes*, it is quite possible that you suffer from insomnia or another sleep disorder.

If you believe that you have a significant sleep problem, then it is likely that you do. Who is a better judge of your own distress than you?

Assuming you are unhappy with your sleep patterns, you have picked up the right book. *Get a Good Night's Sleep* is designed to help you do just what its title says. It explores sleep from both a physiological and a psychological viewpoint. And it offers practical suggestions that will help you rediscover the simple pleasure of a solid night of rest.

(If your employment involves either steady or rotating shift work, then the word *night* in the above paragraphs does not, of course, refer to the literal night. If you must sleep during the day, then your "night" is someone else's "day." For convenience, throughout most of the book I will use the unmodified word *night* to refer to the period of time allotted to you for sleep.)

Sleep Disorders

Data from various sources, including the American Medical Association, suggest that sleep disorders are incredibly common. It is estimated that about one in every three adults suffers from such disorders. In terms of sheer numbers, this is about 60,000,000 people. It is impossible to compute the amount of distress, in forms ranging from auto and industrial accidents to disturbed personal relationships, which arises from problems associated with the loss of sleep.

It is easy to discount the statements of a person who suffers from a sleep disorder. Sometimes the person isn't taken seriously. A husband says to a wife, "I didn't sleep a wink last night." She smiles and says, "Are you kidding? You snored half the night and kept *me* awake. I'm the one who didn't sleep a wink last night." Different people can have very different perceptions of who is and who isn't a good sleeper.

A familiar anecdote, told in various versions, relates the story of a man—let's call him Harry—who complained of insomnia to his physician. At a sleep clinic, Harry was attached to electrodes and viewed on a television monitor. He went promptly to sleep and woke up refreshed almost eight hours later. He admitted that he had never slept more soundly in his life. His complaints were, of course, discounted. Upon reading the clinic's report, his physician laughed and said to himself, "I guess Harry was just imagining things. He doesn't suffer from insomnia at all!"

The sad part of the story is that it is both true and false. Sometimes people with chronic insomnia *do* have a good night of sleep at a clinic, right off the bat, without even having to adapt to the new situation. This seems very odd, doesn't it? It only appears peculiar until you have a better understanding of the nature of sleep.

Harry suffered from a kind of insomnia known as *conditioned insomnia*. Conditioning is a phenomenon of learning. Cues set off involuntary learned responses called *conditioned reflexes*. And these are acquired by association. The fact is that Harry was *negatively* conditioned to the stimuli of his bedroom. In familiar surroundings, he was cued to stay awake. In a different setting, without the usual cues, he was actually able to relax and fall asleep without difficulty. Consequently, Harry *does* have insomnia. But his problem is not physiological in nature. It has no organic basis. It is a problem that is *behavioral*, meaning one that arises from psychological and emotional processes.

People like Harry must be taken seriously. *Anyone* who has a sleep complaint must be taken seriously. A *symptom* is something that *you* experience. It tells you that something is wrong somewhere. And a symptom should never be discounted or ignored.

As you explore the alternative strategies presented in *Get a Good Night's Sleep* for dealing with your own sleep problem, it will be helpful to become familiar with the basic sleep disorders. The identification of these disorders has arisen from both clinical and experimental work conducted in such fields of study as neurology, psychiatry, and psychology.

INSOMNIA

Insomnia is the great wastebasket category. Almost everybody knows the word. You will find it used somewhere in the write-ups printed on almost every over-the-counter box of sleeping pills. In popular usage, almost any sleep disorder earns the quick label of "insomnia."

At a more formal level, *insomnia* is a disorder characterized by one or more of the following symptoms: (1) difficulty in falling asleep; (2) waking up in the middle of the night and then finding it hard to go back to sleep; and (3) waking up too early in the morning. (These three symptoms were used to construct the opening questions of this chapter.)

The word *insomnia* itself is derived from the Latin root *somnus*, meaning sleep. The combining form *in* means "without." So the literal meaning of insomnia is "without sleep."

It is possible to identify two basic kinds of insomnia: (1) symptomatic insomnia and (2) behavioral insomnia.

Symptomatic insomnia is insomnia that is secondary to a medical problem. The insomnia is not a primary disorder in itself, but is a reflection of an underlying organic disturbance. Consequently, the insomnia cannot be successfully treated directly. It will diminish only if the primary physical problem responds to treatment. Examples of conditions that may cause or aggravate symptomatic insomnia include allergies, heart disease, emphysema (which makes it difficult to breathe), rheumatoid arthritis, an enlarged prostate gland (which requires frequent urination during the night), and dependence on medications that interfere with sleep. Alcoholism can also induce insomnia because abuse of alcohol during the day can interfere with normal patterns of sleep at night.

Behavioral insomnia is insomnia that is primary in nature. It *is* the problem. Consequently, it responds to direct treatment. Behavioral insomnia is linked to psychological factors. These include motivational dispositions, learned responses, thought processes, and emotional reactions. When such processes are disturbed, the result is insomnia.

Conditioned insomnia, the kind of insomnia described earlier in connection with Harry, the man who slept soundly in a clinic, is a kind of behavioral insomnia.

Behavioral insomnia can be acute or chronic. If it is *acute*, it is a passing problem. It can be expected to resolve itself without any particular intervention. If insomnia is *chronic*, it tends to go on and on. It may last for months or years.

Chronic behavioral insomnia is the primary subject of this book. It accounts for the vast majority of sleep complaints. It is the kind of insomnia that sends people searching for a new sleeping pill or a new physician. And, fortunately, it is the kind of insomnia that responds well to self-directed coping strategies. It is a miserable condition. But it is not a hopeless one.

SLEEP APNEA

Sleep apnea refers to a series of breathing stops during the night. If respirations completely stop, with substantial frequency, for ten seconds or more during sleep, the individual is likely to suffer from apnea. People with sleep apnea *don't* have insomnia. They seldom complain of tossing and turning during the night. However, they are frequently tired or drowsy during the day, suggesting that they are experiencing significant sleep deprivation. Another sign of sleep apnea is loud snoring. Even infants can suffer from sleep apnea. This is particularly true during the first three months of life when the brain and nervous system are not yet stable in their action. Sleep apnea is thought to be a causal factor in some cases of *sudden infant death syndrome* (SIDS).

A husband or a wife is often the first person to detect sleep apnea in a partner. If your spouse suggests that you snore loudly during the night or that you stop breathing, you should discuss the symptoms with your physician. Although sleep apnea is not in general thought of as a disorder that responds to self-directed interventions, it should be pointed out that a large number of cases of sleep apnea in adults are associated with obesity. Obesity causes fatty deposits toward the base of the tongue that may interfere with sleep. (Crudely put, the individual is choking on fat.) So a good first step if you suspect that you suffer from sleep apnea, and if you are also too heavy, is to make a rational effort to reduce your weight.

HYPERSOMNIA

Hypersomnia is, in a sense, the logical opposite of insomnia. Instead of being unable to fall asleep, the individual finds it difficult to stay awake. In *Type I hypersomnia* the individual falls asleep easily at night. Sometimes this happens early in the evening or, inappropriately, while socializing. The individual appears to sleep soundly most of the night, often finding it difficult to get up in the morning. The victim is somewhat drowsy all day, particularly in the afternoon starting about one o'clock and ending about four o'clock. Hypersomnia, like insomnia, can have medical causes such as a chronic infection, hypoglycemia (low blood sugar), hypothyroidism, narcolepsy (see below), sleep apnea, and anemia. In such cases the hypersomnia can be designated as *symptomatic hypersomnia*. On the other hand, the hypersomnia can arise from an emotional problem such as depression. Another possibility is an unconscious desire to escape from a boring environment. In these cases the proper identification would be *behavioral hypersomnia*.

Type II hypersomnia is a reaction to nighttime insomnia. After an unsettled night, the individual is poorly rested. Consequently, he or she is both tired and sleepy during the day. So it is quite definitely possible for a person to suffer from both insomnia and hypersomnia during a given twenty-four-hour cycle.

NARCOLEPSY

Narcolepsy is characterized by involuntary sleep episodes during the day. The individual suddenly falls asleep for a brief period of time, and this may happen several times a day. Sometimes instead of falling asleep the individual retains consciousness, but loses muscle tone; he or she goes limp and cannot voluntarily sit up properly. This condition is called *cataplexy*. The person may or may not fall asleep right after a bout with cataplexy. There may be *rapid eye movement* (REM) episodes while the person is conscious; normally REM episodes are associated with sleep and dreaming.

Narcolepsy is generally looked upon as a pathological neurological condition, not a psychological one. Consequently, it is usually treated with drug therapy. Drugs may include stimulants and antidepressants. On the behavioral side, the taking of regular naps is recommended.

Although from its name, one might think that narcolepsy is a form of epilepsy, such is not the case. The two conditions should *not* be placed in the same category.

CIRCADIAN RHYTHM SLEEP DISORDER

Circadian rhythm sleep disorder is commonly associated with shift work in which one is required to be on a job at odd hours or on an irregular schedule. Those who work night shifts in hospitals and twenty-four-hour restaurants provide examples of people who might suffer from circadian rhythm sleep disorder.

Jet lag provides another example of circadian rhythm sleep disorder. In general, jet lag appears to be worst when one travels east. The day has to be shortened, and one may find it difficult to fall asleep earlier than usual. A physical clock may say that it is 11:00 P.M. But your biological clock says that it is still only 9:00 P.M. And your biological clock speaks more convincingly than the physical one.

Finally, a third example of circadian rhythm sleep disorder is provided by people who are said to be "larks" and "owls." If you are at your best in the morning, you are a lark. If you are at your best in the evening, you are an owl. Within limits, this is, of course, normal. However, if you are too much of a lark and wake up excessively early, you may lose sleep. In such a case, you are said to have *advanced-phase circadian rhythm sleep disorder*. If you are too much of an owl, and go to bed very late at night, you may also lose sleep. Perhaps you have to get up before you want to in order to get to work on time. In such a case, you are said to have *delayed-phase circadian rhythm sleep disorder*.

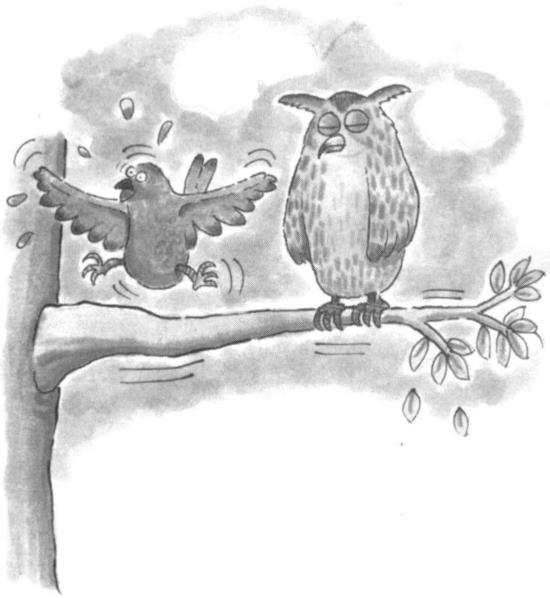

(The word *circadian* comes from Latin roots. *Circa* means "around." *Dies* means "day." Consequently, *circadian* means "around a day.")

PARASOMNIAS

A *parasomnia* is characterized by a significant irregularity during the sleep process. Three parasomnias are

(1) nightmares, (2) night terrors, and (3) and somnambulism. A *nightmare* is a distressing dream. It is associated with REM sleep. One usually wakes up immediately following a nightmare, remembers its details, feels anxious, and often finds it difficult to go back to sleep.

A *night terror* commonly has little content. It is associated with deep sleep. One wakes up bewildered and in a state of near panic without knowing why. Although adults can and do suffer from night terrors, they are more common in children.

Somnambulism is also known as sleepwalking. The individual may have his or her eyes open and do something that appears to require thought, such as take a shower or start dressing. If spoken to gently, there may be a mumbled half-meaningful reply. But the person is clearly asleep. Consequently, the individual is sometimes in danger of bodily injury.

What This Book Can Do for You

If you suffer from insomnia or one of the other sleep disorders, you will find this book useful in several ways.

First, *Get a Good Night's Sleep* will help you decide in your own case whether you suffer from a sleep disorder with a biological basis or a behavioral one.

If your sleep problems have a biological basis, you will be guided in the direction of responsible medical treatment. What you can do for yourself will also be indicated.

If the basis of your problem is behavioral, you will be provided with specific self-directed strategies that will help you correct the difficulty.

This book offers hope. No matter what kind of sleep problem you have, it is probably amenable to treatment. You don't have to continue suffering.

Get a Good Night's Sleep also offers you a sense of self-control. It helps to undercut the awful feeling that you are a victim of adverse forces beyond your control. The vast majority of sleep complaints fall into the general category of behavioral insomnia, which we might also call "common garden-variety insomnia." And behavioral insomnia responds readily to personal interventions.

And finally, you will find specific self-directed strategies clearly identified in a distinctive typeface in the majority of chapters to follow. The strategies are designed to be practical and useful. They are options that you can put to immediate good use in your efforts to neutralize insomnia. Look upon this book as a practical manual.

The Last Word

Sleep, like eating, is a natural process. It might seem odd that a natural process is subject to so many potential disturbances. To a person who does not suffer from insomnia, most of another person's complaints are discounted. "What could be easier than putting you head on the pillow, going to sleep, and getting a sound night of rest?" the skeptic mentally asks.

However, no natural process in human beings is entirely free of disturbance. Think about eating, for example. People have all sorts of gastrointestinal complaints. They suffer from indigestion, gas, constipation, and bowel irritation. Over-the-counter medications for gastrointestinal complaints are right up there on the shelf of your local pharmacy along with medications for sleep.

So insomnia and the sleep disorders must be taken seriously. They are real. And they make people suffer. If you are one of these people, you don't have to be a helpless victim. There is much that can be done for you, and much that you can do for yourself.

Key Points to Remember

- It is estimated that about one in every three Americans suffers from a sleep disorder.
- Anyone who has a sleep complaint must be taken seriously.
- *Insomnia* is a disorder characterized by one or more of the following symptoms: (1) difficulty in falling asleep; (2) waking up in the middle of the night, and then finding it hard to go back to sleep; and (3) waking up too early in the morning.
- *Symptomatic insomnia* is insomnia that is secondary to a medical problem.
- *Behavioral insomnia* is insomnia that is primary in nature. *Conditioned insomnia* is a kind of behavioral insomnia.
- *Chronic behavioral insomnia* is the primary subject of this book.
- *Sleep apnea* refers to a series of breathing stops during the night.
- *Hypersomnia* is characterized by difficulty in staying awake.
- *Narcolepsy* is characterized by involuntary sleep episodes during the day.
- *Circadian rhythm sleep disorder* is commonly associated with shift work and jet lag. It is also associated with people who are "larks" and "owls."
- A *parasomnia* is characterized by a significant irregularity during the sleep process. Three

parasomnias are (1) nightmares; (2) night terrors; and (3) somnambulism, or sleepwalking.

Get a Good Night's Sleep can help you in more than one way. It provides you with useful information concerning sleep and the sleep disorders. Also, it presents a group of specific self-directed strategies that will help you neutralize chronic behavioral insomnia.

2 UNDERSTANDING A NORMAL SLEEP PATTERN: FROM DEEP SLEEP TO LIGHT SLEEP AND BACK AGAIN

It will help you in your quest for future nights of sound sleep to become familiar with the characteristics of a normal sleep pattern. Also, it is useful to know something about the biological processes that control sleep.

This chapter will present some basic information concerning the nature of sleep. In addition, it will present ways in which you can apply that information.

Sleep has been called a "little death." The ego, the conscious self, seems to go into a state of oblivion. We sometimes say of persons in deep sleep, "They are dead to the world." But sleep is not anything like death. In fact, it is a *living process* with a complex set of attributes.

Throughout the centuries sleep has been looked upon as mysterious. Many prescientific cultures hold the idea that the soul leaves the body during sleep and travels into other realms—to the stars or other dimensions. Again, there is the danger of death—the soul in its journeying might get lost or might not be able to reenter the body. These ideas probably arise from the experience of dreams. Instead of thinking of dreams as mental phenomena, uninformed persons think that perhaps dreams reflected real experiences of some sort.

Most of the myth and folklore about sleeping and dreaming is based on a mystical viewpoint. In this book we will take a different viewpoint, that of natural science.

The general value of this viewpoint is that *you* take control of behavioral events. In order to do this, you need to have access to the key findings of contemporary research.

Stages of Sleep

Research conducted by Wilse B. Webb and others has revealed that there are several stages of sleep. These are designated as follows: Stage 0, Stage 1, Stage 2, Stage 3, and Stage 4.

Stage 0 is not sleep at all. It is a label useful as a device for classifying data in experimental work. It is not really meaningful to speak of Stage 0 sleep. However, one might speak of Stage 0 consciousness, using this designation to refer to a presleep stage in which one's consciousness is diffuse, as it sometimes is during meditation. During Stage 0 many of us, not all, are prone to odd dreamlike impressions and images that appear unbidden, probably from an unconscious level of the mind. The name given to this aspect of Stage 0 consciousness is *hypnagogic reverie*. (*Hypno* is a combining form meaning sleep. In Greek mythology, the god of sleep is Hypnos.)

Stage 1 sleep is borderline sleep. We use terms such as *drowsy* or *light sleep* to capture its essence. Jerking muscles are sometimes associated with this stage. Off and on, about 5 percent to 10 percent of a typical night is spent in Stage 1.

Stage 2 sleep is genuine sleep. It is a stepping stone to deeper stages.

Stage 3 sleep is relatively deep sleep. If an electroencephalographic (EEG) recording is made of a person in Stage 3, long, slow wave patterns will begin to appear at the rate of about four cycles per second. These are called *delta waves*.

Stage 4 sleep is the deepest stage of sleep. The delta waves become very pronounced. Evidence suggests that the body is restoring itself. The sleep is profound and dreamless. People in Stage 4 sleep are difficult to awaken.

All of the stages described above refer to *nonrapid eye movement (NREM) sleep*. If a person is awakened during NREM sleep, he or she will seldom report a dream.

There is another kind of sleep. It is called *rapid eye movement (REM) sleep*. If a person is awakened during a REM episode, he or she will usually report a well-defined dream.

REM sleep obtains its name from the fact that during this kind of sleep an observer can actually see the eyeballs moving rapidly, seemingly at random, below the eyelids. It is as if the person is looking at a motion picture. This, of course, suggests a connection with the visual experiences that we are likely to have when we dream.

REM sleep is associated with light sleep. Sometimes it is called Stage I REM. The average adult spends about 20 percent to 25 percent of a typical night in REM sleep. If an EEG recording is made during REM sleep, the waves will have a rate of about fourteen cycles per second. The tracings will be "busy" and complex. In fact, it is difficult to see much difference between the EEG tracings obtained when a person is in REM sleep and those obtained when a person is in a normal waking state. For this reason, REM sleep is sometimes called "paradoxical sleep."

The entire sleep cycle will repeat itself five, six, or even seven times during the night depending on the individual and the total duration of sleep.

Infants sleep about sixteen hours in every twenty-four-hour period. And they spend about 50 percent of that time in REM sleep. Going to the other end of the scale in terms of chronological age, elderly people tend to sleep less than young adults. Six and one-half hours of sleep can be quite normal and restorative to a person who is over sixty years of age. The time spent in REM sleep will be equivalent to adults in general, about 20 percent to 25 percent.

Making Applications

With a knowledge of the sleep cycle and the existence of NREM and REM sleep, it is possible to make some meaningful applications. This section presents self-directed strategies that have a logical connection to the facts presented in the prior section.

A POSITIVE ATTITUDE

Take the Positive Attitude That Time Spent Sleeping Is Time Well Spent. Sometimes insomnia is aggravated by the negative attitude that sleep is a waste of time. Benjamin Franklin gave this advice: "Up, sluggard, and waste not life; in the grave will be sleeping enough."

And it is sometimes said that Thomas Alva Edison developed the lightbulb because he thought that the gift of consciousness should not be wasted. With artificial light, he reasoned, sleep was hardly necessary. Biographical sketches of Edison often indicate that he did not believe in sleeping for a sustained period of time. Instead, he took fifteen- to twenty-minute catnaps on a couch in his laboratory at any time of the day or night.

In spite of the attitudes expressed by Franklin and Edison, a wealth of data suggest that sleep is necessary. (And, after all, both Franklin and Edison did in fact sleep.) It refreshes the body, helps it to rebuild and repair its cells, and even recharges the immune system. People who are chronically sleep deprived suffer from fatigue and may even be more prone to infections than others.

Experiments with rats indicate that if they are forced to stay awake for prolonged periods of time, they die. Apparently the stress of gross sleep deprivation overwhelms the body's adaptive resources. What is true of rats is quite likely to be true of human beings.

Experiments with human beings are, of course, not carried as far as with rats. But it has been found that human beings who are systematically deprived of sleep become disoriented. Their thinking may become delusional and their moods become erratic.

Sleep is a biological need. Don't fight it.

SLEEP AND THE WILL

Recognize That Sleep Is Not Under the Direct Control of the Will. There is no point in trying to will yourself to go to sleep because you can't do it. Here's a personal experiment you can conduct. Will the pupil of your eye to dilate, to get larger and admit more light. Go look at yourself in a bathroom mirror and try it. Nothing happens in response to your will. Now turn off the room light. You will see your pupil automatically dilate. You have controlled the dilation *indirectly*. Turning off the light switch was an action that you were able to will.

Similarly, sleep is like the pupillary reflex. It cannot be directly controlled. But there are actions, plenty of them, that you *can* will that will *induce* sleep. And there is a key word. *Induce.* The art of sleeping well is the art of sleep induction. The many suggestions and skills presented in this book are actions under your direct control. They are the gateways that make the inevitable induction of sleep possible.

It is useless to toss and turn and repeatedly say to yourself, "Go to sleep." You must not give yourself direct commands of this kind. Paradoxically, they tend to keep you on alert and inhibit sleep.

You can't *force* yourself to go to sleep. The art of sleep induction is a gentle art. Say this to yourself: "I can go to sleep easily by learning how to *induce* sleep."

MELATONIN AND SLEEP

Help Your Body Produce Melatonin. The seventeenth-century philosopher René Descartes suggested that the pineal gland is the point where the soul interacts with the body. The pineal gland is located in the brain and is not

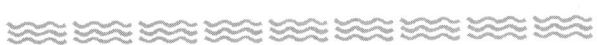

much larger than the head of a pin. Today Descartes's observation is usually dismissed as quaint. Interestingly, it has overtones of the ancient belief that the soul departs the body during sleep. And it turns out that the pineal gland *does* play an important role in sleep. So perhaps Descartes was moving in the right general direction.

Contemporary research suggests that the pineal gland regulates circadian rhythms. It manages to do this by secreting a hormone called *melatonin*. Melatonin, a chemical messenger, has an impact on specific clusters of neurons in the brain that "turn on" sleep. A reduction of light levels in the external world is the cue that activates the pineal gland to increase its secretion of melatonin. Conversely, high light levels inhibit the secretion of melatonin.

However, it is important to realize that high light levels during the day help the body to manufacture melatonin. The ideal formula for melatonin production is this: Plenty of natural, full-spectrum light during the day and ample darkness at night. The more you can approximate this ideal, the more you will encourage your pineal gland to first generate and then secrete optimal amounts of melatonin.

From a practical point of view, here are some things you can do to take advantage of the action of melatonin.

1. If you work in an artificial light environment, try to get some natural sunlight during the day. Even a daily twenty-minute walk outdoors will be helpful.

2. Work with as much light as possible. Use indirect light that does not glare and cause eye strain. But *do* keep the ambient light level high. For example, if you work at a computer, and you have any control over your environment, be sure that there is ample surrounding light.

3. When you go to bed, make sure that the room is as dark as possible. If you have a lighted clock on

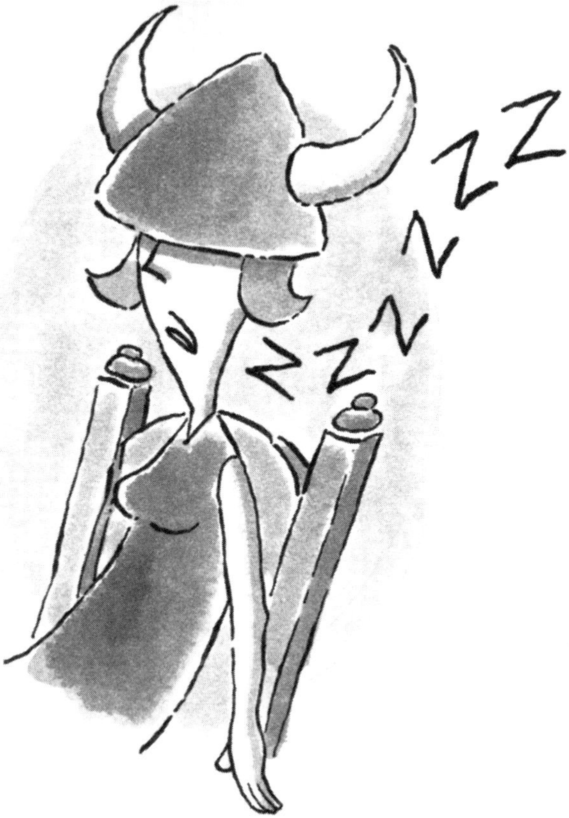

your bed stand, remove it from your visual field. A small, indirect night light will probably not interfere with melatonin production. But allow no more ambient light than this.

4. Make sure that your windows admit little or no light in the morning. If, for example, you have sheer drapes, line them with an opaque material that will not admit outside light. This will keep you from waking up too early.

5. Don't shock your pineal gland with a burst of light. If you must use the bathroom during the night, do it by a dim night light. When you go into the bathroom, turn on the switch, and flood your eyes with light, you inhibit the action of the pineal gland. It will, for a while, stop producing melatonin. You might find it hard to return to sleep when you go back to bed. An alternative to a night light is to equip your bathroom with a dimmer switch. Have it preset in a dim position so that when you turn it on you will obtain only the minimal light that you need.

6. If you are doing shift work and must sleep during the day in a room with too much ambient light, consider wearing a sleep mask. Such a mask is opaque, and from the point of view of your eyes and your brain, it will be as if you are in a dark room. The only problem—and it *is* a problem for some people—is adapting to the mask. Anything that is new tends to increase arousal and interfere with sleep. So you do have to make up your mind to get used to the mask. Assuming you can do this, it can really be helpful in helping your pineal gland produce melatonin and give you a full seven or eight hours of rest.

What about taking melatonin supplements? These are available in health food stores. It is asserted that these can possibly not only help you sleep, but even slow down the aging process. It is too early to assess the various claims for melatonin sold in bottled form. There is no scientific consensus except the consensus to use common sense and proceed with caution. Although melatonin is a natural substance, no one knows for sure what are the long-term side effects of taking it for prolonged periods. At present, the most prudent advice appears to be to avoid using melatonin supplements on a regular basis. However, they may be helpful in coping with circadian rhythm disorder, including jet lag.

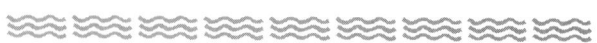

SEROTONIN AND SLEEP

Help Your Body Produce Serotonin. Serotonin is another key chemical messenger involved in sleep. The neurons in your brain and nervous system naturally manufacture serotonin. If serotonin levels are low, this is likely to interfere with sleep. In order to help your body to produce optimal amounts of needed serotonin, there are three practical actions you can easily take.

First, restrict your intake of refined sugar. This is simple table sugar, or sucrose. The problem is not so much the sugar you spoon directly into a cup of coffee or other beverage. The real difficulty arises from the fact that many of our foods contain sugar. This is called *hidden sugar*. The list of such foods is long and includes cake, pie, cookies, ice cream, candy, jelly, jam, doughnuts, syrup, and more. Various studies suggest that the average adult consumes about two pounds of sugar a week. (Adolescents consume about three pounds of sugar a week.)

It requires B-complex vitamins to break table sugar down into blood glucose. Consequently, if you eat a diet that is too high in sugar, you may induce a B-complex deficiency. The B-complex vitamins are required in order to manufacture serotonin. Consequently, there is a domino effect. A B-complex deficiency may be a causal factor associated with low levels of serotonin. And low levels of serotonin make it difficult to sleep.

Second, eat foods containing high levels of the amino acid *tryptophan*. Foods high in this amino acid include beef, poultry, fish, milk, cheese, eggs, legumes, and leafy green vegetables. Turkey and milk appear to be particularly high in tryptophan. Tryptophan is a key ingredient used by neurons to manufacture serotonin.

However, the tryptophan picture is not quite as clear as it was once thought to be. Relatively recent research suggests that high-protein foods have the net effect of blocking much of the available tryptophan that reaches the brain. It is possible that eating carbohydrates may assist the transport system that carries tryptophan to the

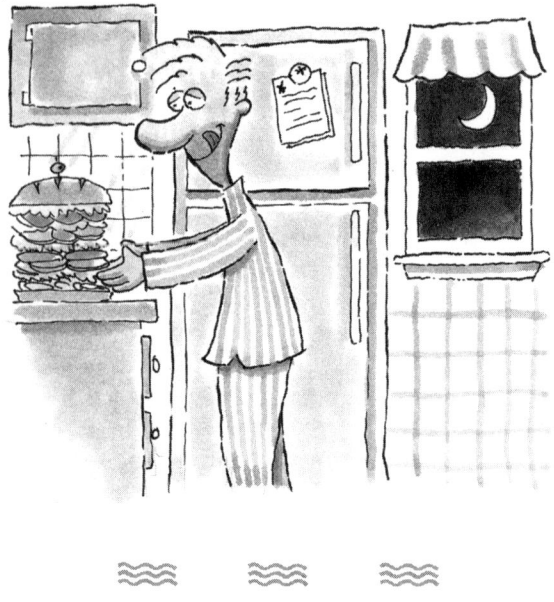

brain. Consequently, it might be better to eat a slice of toast along with a slice of turkey as a sleep-inducing snack, instead of eating two slices of turkey. Green vegetables are also of particular value because they are low in protein and high in carbohydrate.

What about supplemental tryptophan in tablet form? Research suggests that excessive tryptophan in this form is sometimes linked to a blood disorder in which there are too many white blood cells. This is a dangerous condition. Consequently, it is generally recommended that one *not* take supplemental tryptophan. Get your tryptophan from food, its natural source. There's plenty of it available in the items on the list provided.

Third, you can eat foods rich in B-complex vitamins. Here is a list of foods rich in these vitamins:

Avocados

Bananas

Beef, poultry, and fish

Bran

Brewer's yeast

Brown rice

Bulgar wheat

Eggs

Leafy green vegetables

Legumes

Milk

Molasses

Nuts (particularly peanuts, which in fact are a kind of legume)

Soybeans

Wheat germ

Whole grain bread

Take note of the fact that many of the foods high in B-complex vitamins also are high in tryptophan. So you get a bonus from eating these foods. If your daily diet is low in the above foods, you may have low levels of serotonin. And this may be one reason you find it difficult to sleep.

If you don't get enough B-complex vitamins from your food, or if you ingest too much sugar, you might want to consider taking a B-complex supplement. These are readily available in drug stores, supermarkets, and health food stores. It is, of course, better to get your vitamins from your food. If you do decide to take a supplement, be sure you take it with a certain amount of caution: Some vitamins, particularly oil-based ones such as vitamins A, D, and E, can be toxic if taken in large doses. In general, however, the B-complex vitamins do not tend to be toxic.

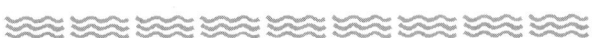

SLEEPING PILLS

Use Sleeping Pills on a Highly Limited Basis, If at All. The answer to sleep does not reside in a box or bottle of pills.

Drugs that induce sleep include antihistamines, antianxiety agents, and barbiturates. Some of these are available over the counter; others require a prescription.

There are several problems associated with the use of sleeping pills. First, they may in some cases be *physiologically addictive*. This makes it difficult to withdraw from them without symptoms such as headaches, cramps, or shakiness. Second, they are quite likely to be *psychologically addictive*. This means that even if your body does not actually demand the drug, you become emotionally dependent on it. It becomes a psychological crutch that you hate to give up. Third, all drugs are to some degree toxic and may have adverse side effects.

Fourth, and perhaps most important in terms of sleep, sleep-inducing drugs may interfere with REM sleep. Drugs tend to increase the amount of deep, NREM sleep. The consequence of this is that you may be deprived of some of your dreaming time. This is a very significant loss because a large body of clinical and experimental evidence suggests that you *need to dream* in order to maintain your mental health. (There will be more about dreaming in Chapter 4.)

Most boxes of over-the-counter sleeping pills contain the warning that the contents are to be used for *occasional* insomnia. Clearly, they are not a treatment for chronic insomnia. If a transient situation is making you worried, or if you are suffering from jet lag, or if some other passing problem is adversely affecting your sleep, then sleeping pills might be justified for a few days.

ALCOHOL

Avoid Using Alcohol as a Sleeping Potion. It was fashionable for physicians in England some years ago to prescribe to elderly patients who complained of insomnia that they take a "bit of port" before going to bed. Port wine is a sweet wine containing about 20 percent alcohol. Two ounces of such wine is equivalent to a one-ounce shot of 80-proof whiskey. (The proof content is equivalent to double the actual alcohol content.)

Whether you obtain your alcohol from sweet wine, dry wine, beer, whiskey, or other alcoholic beverage, the influence of alcohol on the brain and nervous system is about the same (depending on the amount ingested). Alcohol is a central nervous depressant. It *will* help you to fall asleep. However, research suggests that alcohol may interfere with the entire range of the nightly sleep pattern. You may, for example, only experience three or four of the individual cycles instead of five or six. Roy E., a retired sixty-seven-year-old engineer, says, "I tried drinking a little wine just before I went to bed. It helped me to go to sleep quickly. But I found I was waking up around two or three o'clock every morning. And I couldn't get back to sleep. So I quit the alcoholic nightcap." Roy's experience is not uncommon.

VENTILATION

Be Sure Your Bedroom Is Well Ventilated. Two of the structures in your brain stem are called the *pons* and the *medulla*. Working together, they regulate breathing. They contain neurons that are capable of reading carbon dioxide (CO_2) levels in your blood. When you inhale, you use up oxygen. Your body constantly uses oxygen to sustain its overall metabolic process. When you exhale, the breath you return to the environment is high in carbon dioxide; it is a waste product of metabolism. Consequently, in a completely closed room, you would eventually suffocate: You would use up all of the oxygen, and you would have nothing but nonusable carbon dioxide left.

In a room in which the carbon dioxide levels are gradually rising, your pons and medulla will compensate by sending messages down the spinal cord to your diaphragm. These messages say, "Breathe more rapidly. Take in more oxygen." Your respirations will automatically increase without an act of will on your part. You may or may not be conscious of the increase in rate. If the increase is moderate, you may not notice it. If the increase is significant, you will probably be aware that you are breathing rapidly.

In a poorly ventilated room your respirations may increase from an initial resting state of twelve to fourteen a minute to perhaps eighteen or twenty a minute. Let's say that you retire at 11:00 P.M. in a poorly ventilated room. By 3:00 A.M. you have used up a significant amount of oxygen. You are breathing rapidly. A rapid rate of breathing is associated with high central nervous system arousal. Subconsciously, this is perceived as excitement. Anything that excites you is antagonistic to sleep. You are very likely to wake up and find yourself in a state of vigilance, a state that will make it difficult to relax and go back to sleep.

ROOM TEMPERATURE

Be Sure That the Room Temperature Is Comfortable. If a room is too cold, and if you are inadequately covered, you may shiver and shake a little. This increases central nervous system arousal, puts you on alert, and makes it difficult to either go to sleep or sustain sleep. On the other hand, if you are too warm, you will feel uncomfortable too. You may sweat excessively and throw off the blankets.

There are host of practical considerations that may make it difficult for you to ensure that the bedroom's temperature is comfortable. For example, if you don't have an air-conditioning system in your home, you may be forced to sleep in a too warm room. This, of course, is why screened sleeping porches were popular a number of years ago.

Within realistic limits, do your best to either seek or produce an optimal temperature. A room temperature of about sixty-five degrees is ideal for many people. Five degrees above or below this average is also often perceived as comfortable.

The Last Word

Sleep is both a physiological and a psychological process. This chapter has focused on the physiological aspects of sleep. It presented a description of the normal sleep pattern in human beings.

Although the physiological processes associated with sleep are under involuntary control, the conditions that induce these processes are responsive to your voluntary actions. Consequently, there is much that you can do to take charge of what happens to you at a biological level when you sleep. The self-directed strategies in this chapter showed you practical ways in which this goal can be accomplished. The strategies are simple and can be readily applied. Use them, and the duration and quality of your sleep will gradually improve.

Key Points to Remember

- The stages of sleep are: Stage 0, Stage 1, Stage 2, Stage 3, and Stage 4.
- In addition to the stages, a distinction is made between *nonrapid eye movement (NREM)* sleep and *rapid eye movement (REM)* sleep. REM sleep is associated with dreaming
- Take the positive attitude that time spent sleeping is time well spent.
- Recognize that sleep is not under the direct control of the will.

- Help your body produce melatonin.
- Help your body produce serotonin.
- Use sleeping pills on a highly limited basis, if at all.
- Avoid using alcohol as a sleeping potion.
- Be sure your bedroom is well ventilated.
- Be sure that the room temperature is comfortable.

3 EMOTIONS AND SLEEP: BLUES IN THE NIGHT

Natalie L. is a thirty-eight-year-old married woman with four children. She lives with her husband and her children in a pleasant suburb. Her three-thousand-square-foot house is surrounded by a lush lawn. Natalie is a full-time homemaker, a loving wife, and an effective mother. She also suffers from chronic behavioral insomnia.

Talking to her family physician, she says, "For me, the Big Bad Wolf that eats the sheep of sleep is anxiety. When I put my head on the pillow I start to worry about bills I have to pay, how the kids are doing in school, and all sorts of similar details surrounding daily living. I'm pretty calm when I get into bed, but then I start thinking. And I get myself going. Pretty soon I'm wide awake and I can tell my pulse has become more rapid. And I'm breathing hard. What can I do?"

Nancy's physician can, of course, prescribe an antianxiety drug. This is a "quick fix" for the problem. It *is* a respectable treatment, but it *is not* a cure. There is much Nancy can do for herself to cope with nighttime anxiety. And if you, like Nancy, have a similar problem, the strategies offered in this chapter may be of some assistance.

Actually, the Big Bad Wolf of anxiety is not the only one. Other prominent emotional wolves of the night include anger, guilt, depression, and lovesickness. Let's examine these moods and evaluate what can be done to keep them from robbing you of your sleep.

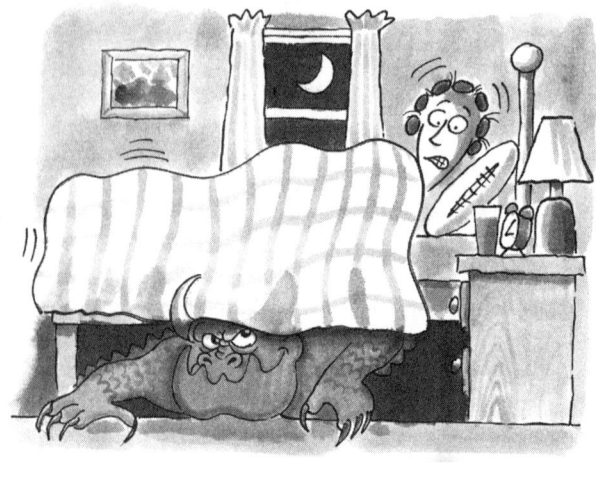

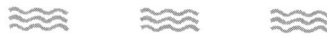

Examining Emotions

What would life be like without emotions? In some ways it would be much better. There would be no sadness, no anger, no unhappiness. We wouldn't *feel* anything.

On the other hand, in some ways life would be much worse. There would be no laughter, no joy, no moments of ecstasy. So the aim of this chapter is *not* to teach you how to eliminate emotions. If you would have the upside of emotions, you must take some of the downside. Nonetheless, it is possible to *modulate* negative emotions to restrict their pathological influence on you. In particular, in the case of sleep, if you can do this you can enjoy more restful nights.

Emotions have two dimensions. The first dimension is called *hedonic tone*. This means that emotions can range from *unpleasant* at one end of a first psychological continuum to *pleasant* at the other end. The second dimension is called *arousal*. This indicates that emotions can range from *calm* at one end of a second psychological continuum to *excitement* at the other end. This way of looking at emotions, inspired by Wilhelm Wundt, the principal founder of experimental psychology, generates four basic categories of emotions:

1. *Unpleasant-calm.* Words used to capture the unpleasant-calm emotional state include *disappointment*, the *"blahs,"* *dejection*, *despair*, *discouragement*, *gloom*, *demoralization*, and *depression*. Because you are, in a sense, calm, an emotional state such as depression may or may not rob you of sleep. However, if you *do* sleep, it will not be a completely restful, natural sleep.

2. *Pleasant-calm.* Words used to capture the pleasant-calm emotional state include *serenity*, *"peace of mind,"* *placidity*, *tranquility*, *equanimity*, and *composure*. This is the ideal emotional state for sleep. It is the one you want to cultivate.

3. *Unpleasant-excitement.* Words used to capture the unpleasant-excitement emotional state include *irritation*, *upset*, *agitation*, *anger*, *rage*, *fury*, *wrath*, *exasperation*, *indignation*, *resentment*, and *hostility*. This is the worst emotional state for sleep. It is very difficult to relax and go to sleep when one is in the grips of an emotion such as anger.

4. *Pleasant-excitement.* Words used to capture the pleasant-excitement emotional state include *cheerful*, *delighted*, *glad*, *elated*, and *ecstatic*. Although it would seem to be desirable to be in a pleasant-excited state, the truth is that if you are too excited, the high level of arousal may interfere with sleep.

Coping with Emotional States

Human beings have a strong general tendency to feel that we are entitled to our emotions. Most of us really detest it when someone attempts to trivialize one of our moods by saying something such as, "Oh, you're being silly," or, "That's just childish on your part." We will not be told by others *what* to feel and *how* to feel.

But how about *you*? How about learning to listen to yourself instead of listening to others? Do you believe that it is possible to reflect on your own thoughts, reevaluate them, and take at least partial charge of your emotional states?

The *cognitive theory* of emotions asserts that it *is* possible to voluntarily modify our own moods to some extent. This is done by *challenging* our unbidden, rather idiosyncratic, thoughts. The psychiatrist Aaron Beck calls these *automatic thoughts*. They arise without reflection, are often irrational, and frequently generate negative emotional states. You can counter an automatic thought with a *voluntary thought*. A voluntary thought is well considered. It is based on reason and intelligence; consequently, it can undercut the adverse effects of automatic thoughts.

WORRY AND ANXIETY

Learn to Look Upon Much of Your Worrying as a Useless Mental Activity That Generates Unnecessary Anxiety. Although *worry* and *anxiety* are sometimes used as more or less synonymous terms, let us, for the sake of convenience, associate worry with the thoughts that you think. And let's associate anxiety with the emotional state generated by these thoughts. This distinction will help us to target the *cause* of your anxiety, your self-defeating thoughts.

Worry is, of course, somewhat natural for human beings. This is because we can anticipate the future. We can project our minds forward in time and imagine the worst. (Note that we can also imagine, if we work at it, the best!) It is important to realize that when we worry we *create* fictional future worlds. The things we worry about haven't happened. They *might* happen. Therefore they are not realities, but figments of our imaginations. They are ghosts that we have conjured up out of our own insecurities.

Here are some examples of automatic thoughts that have caused some of my counseling clients anxiety. Immediately following are examples of voluntary thoughts that can diminish the level of anxiety.

Automatic thoughts: "I've got to get the electricity bill paid first thing tomorrow. Otherwise the company might turn off the power." *Voluntary thoughts*: "The bill is only two days overdue. I'm sure that the company gives at least a two-week grace period. I haven't even received a second notice. I don't have anything to worry about."

Automatic thoughts: "Maybe the batteries in the smoke alarm are dead. I haven't checked them for quite a while. What if there's a fire during the night? Patrick and I and the kids could all be suffocated and die of smoke inhalation." *Voluntary thoughts*: "I'm thirty-eight years old and I've never been in a house fire. The house *might* catch on fire; but it probably *won't*. Maybe the batteries aren't dead. I'll check the smoke alarm first thing tomorrow and get new batteries if it needs them."

Automatic thoughts: "I have a big examination in my math class tomorrow. I'll probably get a D or an F on it. I always do badly in math." *Voluntary thoughts*: "I'm well prepared for the examination. I don't *always* do badly in math. Actually, I got a B and a C on my last two tests."

Automatic thoughts: "I'm being interviewed for a new job tomorrow. I'll probably goof up the interview and make a fool out of myself." *Voluntary thoughts*: "I've been interviewed for jobs several times. When I'm actually in the interview, in spite of my fears, I usually handle myself fairly well. And I've been hired a number of times after I've been interviewed."

Automatic thoughts form themselves. Voluntary thoughts take mental effort. If automatic thoughts are causing you anxiety, and if the voluntary thoughts you try to fashion in bed are inadequate to the task, get up for a few minutes. Go to a quiet place and write out the voluntary thoughts that will neutralize the automatic ones. Then go back to bed and focus on the voluntary thoughts.

Voluntary thoughts that are antagonistic to anxiety-arousing automatic ones act as natural tranquilizers.

ANGER

Take the Viewpoint That Anger Is a Form of Self-Indulgence. The core of anger is self-pity. And the self-pity, if carefully scrutinized, is often *unjustified*.

The psychological chain of events associated with anger begins with a *frustrating event*. There is something you want that you can't get. Or there is something you want to get away from that you can't escape. (Define these concepts very broadly. For example, something you want that you can't get might be a certain kind of behavior on the part of a spouse or your children.)

Then you have a *belief* about the frustrating event. This is the automatic thought. If the belief is somewhat irrational, as it often is, you will then experience anger.

Here are some examples of automatic thoughts that have caused some of my counseling clients anger. Immediately following are examples of voluntary thoughts that can diminish the intensity of the anger.

Automatic thoughts: "Tonight at dinner I tried to tell Alice about the new assignments I've been getting at work. I wanted to share the sense of challenge that they're giving me. But she was more interested in feeding Susan than in listening to me. She always ignores me."
Voluntary thoughts: "Alice has never been to my place of work. It is very hard for her to visualize what I do. I can't expect her to take a lot of interest in something that is just

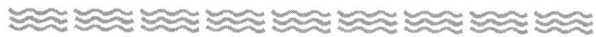

an abstraction to her. And she doesn't *always* ignore me. I remember we had a pretty good conversation about my work just last week. Susan is getting over a cold and Alice is naturally worried about her nutrition."

Automatic thoughts: "Ray never treats me like a sweetheart any more. He takes me for granted all of the time. He comes home late from work without explanation, expects a good meal on the table in a few minutes, and I don't even get a 'thank you.' *Voluntary thoughts*: "I'm oversimplifying our relationship. On our wedding anniversary Ray surprised me with two tickets to a dinner theater performance of *Camelot*. I remember he gave me his undivided attention for the whole evening. So he does *not* take me for granted *all* of the time. He has told me that he will be home late at least two or three nights a week for the next month or so. I can't expect "thank yous" for everyday household responsibilities. I don't usually give him "thank yous" when he washes the car, mows the lawn, or throws out the trash. Maybe *he* feels taken for granted too."

Automatic thoughts: "Shana is unbelievable! Her room is a mess! She never makes her bed properly. She's fat. She's failing all of her classes. And I can't tell her anything." (Shana is sixteen years old, and the thoughts belong to her mother.) *Voluntary thoughts*: "If I'm honest, I probably wasn't much better when I was sixteen. She does in fact make her bed properly when I ask her to straighten up because we're having company. She's about fifteen pounds overweight, but maybe it's an overstatement on my part to call her "fat." She's getting a D in algebra; but I think she's getting a C or better in her other classes. Although she discounts much of what I say, *sometimes* she listen to me when I talk. I'm whipping myself up into a froth. Shana's behavior is neither completely acceptable nor completely unacceptable. She's just an average teenager."

Voluntary thoughts that are antagonistic to anger-arousing automatic ones tend to calm you down and help you to go to sleep.

GUILT

Realize That Much of Your Guilt May Arise from an Overly Strict Superego. If during the presleep interval you are thinking that you are an awful person or that you are to blame for someone else's loss, it will be hard to let go of self-awareness and fall asleep. Guilt involves a high level of *self-monitoring*, a tendency to look at your own behavior too closely.

In classical psychoanalysis, the agent associated with moral self-monitoring is called the *superego*. Freud said that it is the agent of the personality representing your parents in their absence. Assume that your parents were extremely strict and overcontrolling. Also assume that you loved them and that they loved you. Finally, assume that you adopted their value system. Given these conditions, you are likely to have a punitive superego. It rakes you over the coals for even minor infractions of what you "should do" and "shouldn't have done." A punitive superego can't be pleased. You are always a child to it, and you are always in the wrong.

Here are some examples of automatic thoughts that have caused some of my counseling clients to feel guilty. Immediately following are examples of voluntary thoughts that can dispel some of the guilt.

Automatic thoughts: "I lied to my best friend, Margery, today. I told her that I couldn't go out to lunch with her because my mother was coming over to visit. It was an out-and-out falsehood. I just didn't feel like getting myself put together for one more chitchat luncheon. But I'm ashamed of myself for feeling this way. Margery is always there for me. She sticks with me through thick or thin. And she deserves better treatment from her best friend."
Voluntary thoughts: "I was told by my mother to never tell a lie, even a little lie. And I think that my guilt is mainly coming from my mother's teachings, teachings I've never really examined objectively. Actually, I told Margery the lie *not* for myself, but for her. I told it to spare her feelings. Maybe ideally I should have been more honest in

some way. But I didn't hurt Margery. And I *do* care about her. And I *will* make it up to her. So I don't really have all that much to feel guilty about."

Automatic thoughts: "I can't believe it. Today I called my husband, the man I love, a fool. I could see the hurt on his face. I promised myself on the day I got married that I wouldn't indulge in name calling. And now I've broken my promise to myself. I'm more of a fool than he is." *Voluntary thoughts*: "Today he lost $200 at the racetrack, money we can ill afford to lose. He certainly is *not* a fool because he does many wise and prudent things. But his gambling *behavior* was foolish, and deserves to be so labeled. I'm not going to call him a fool again, because he isn't one. But I'm certainly going to call foolish actions by their right name. I think I can forgive myself this one time because I was so taken aback by what he did."

Automatic thoughts: "Today I had a vivid sexual fantasy involving Sallyann. This goes completely against everything I believe in. Colleen is a faithful, sexually responsive wife. And she deserves better than this. If she could read my mind, she would be disgusted with me." (Sallyann is a coworker.) *Voluntary thoughts*: "The sexual fantasy thrust itself on me unbidden. I didn't want it; it just happened. And I have no intention of ever acting on it in any way. I'm not going to flirt with Sallyann or display the least bit of visible erotic interest. As long as I don't act on my impulses, I don't have anything to feel guilty about. And Colleen *can't* read minds. Nobody can. So I can relax on that account."

Voluntary thoughts that are antagonistic to guilt-producing automatic ones can help you relax and settle down.

DEPRESSION

Put the Day's Disappointments Into a Larger Perspective. Depression has a somewhat unpredictable effect on sleep. On the one hand, if a person suffers from a significant chronic depression, the result may by hypersomnia.

The individual may sleep too long and too frequently in an unconscious effort to escape the misery of life. On the other hand, if depression is mild and transient, if it is related to a disappointment suffered during the day, it can rob one of sleep. It is this second type of depression, a transient mood state experienced by us all, that often responds promptly to appropriate voluntary thoughts.

Here are some examples of automatic thoughts that have caused some of my counseling clients to feel depressed. Immediately following are examples of voluntary thoughts that can remove some of the gloom.

Automatic thoughts: "I got a D on my history examination. One more D like that and I'll get a D in the course. There is no way that I can graduate from college if I keep up this kind of thing. Maybe it's all hopeless. What's a person my age with two kids doing trying to go back to school anyway? If I just drop out and concentrate on making a living, life would be a lot easier." (The thinker is a twenty-seven-year-old divorced mother of two children. She works thirty hours a week as a waitress and goes to a local community college as a part-time student. Her goal is to become a registered nurse.) *Voluntary thoughts*: "Even if I *do* get a D in the course, it won't be a disaster. The school will let me repeat a D or an F grade for a higher one. So I'll have a second chance. My overall average is a B. I'm really doing very well considering I'm the sole breadwinner for my family. And I'm getting an A in anatomy and physiology, a course that really counts in my prenursing program. I'm going to make it. I *will* make it. I just have to stick to it and believe in myself."

Automatic thoughts: "The manuscript for my novel just came back with a form rejection letter for the fourth time. It's probably worthless, a piece of junk. What makes me think I can write salable fiction anyway? I don't get any encouragement from anyone. My girlfriend thinks I'm wasting my time and lets me know it. Maybe I don't have any talent." *Voluntary thoughts*: "Most authors had to endure quite a bit of rejection before they sold a manuscript. Many good books are returned for no particular reason. Eventually I'll capture someone's attention with my book if I just keep submitting it. I've got to believe in myself."

Automatic thoughts: "Our offer on the house was turned down. And it's a pretty bitter pill to swallow. I had my heart set on that house. I can just see me and Craig and the children in it. I would be just perfect. I've got to get out of this rented apartment. It's small and ugly and it's stifling my soul." *Voluntary thoughts*: "Although the offer was turned down, I'm sure we'll have one accepted eventually. It doesn't make sense to set my heart on a particular house until escrow actually closes. The apartment is clean and decent and will do until we can move. The important thing to remember is that home is where the heart is."

LOVESICKNESS

Recognize That Lovesickness Has Its Origins in Idealization. In Irving Berlin's musical play *Call Me Madam* one particular song expresses the idea that the hero tosses in his sleep at night. He is told that he isn't sick; he's just in love. Put the words *sick* and *love* together and you create the word *lovesickness*. One standard dictionary defines lovesickness as "languishing with love."

In general, lovesickness tends to occur when one person projects impossible attributions and unrealistic expectations on another person. The pathology is intensified if there is little or any hope of having the love returned. Dorian has a crush on Nina. He thinks she's the cutest thing he's ever seen. But he never tells her and has no real hope that his feelings toward her can ever take a realistic turn. Dorian is lovesick.

Here are some examples of automatic thoughts that have caused some of my counseling clients to be lovesick. Immediately following are examples of voluntary thoughts that can make the individual feel better.

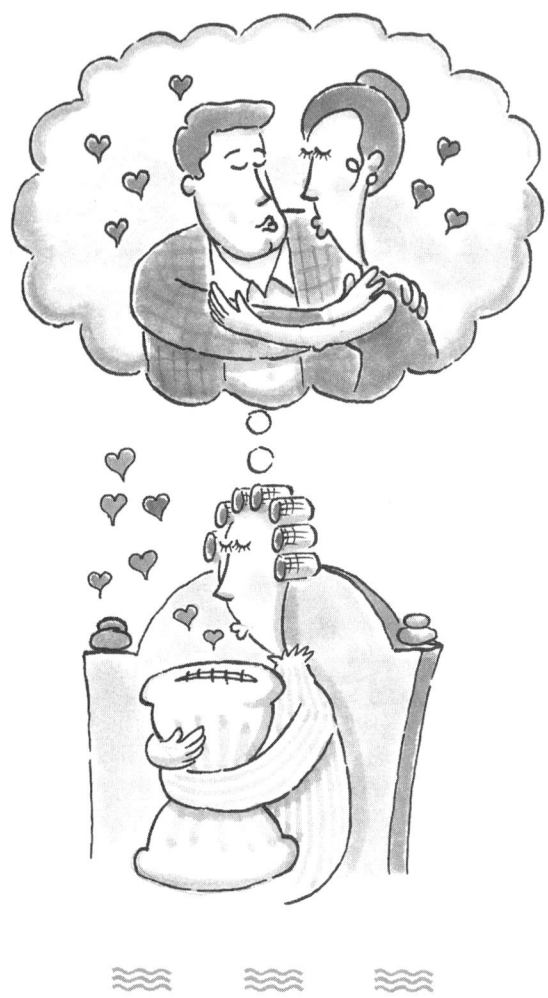

Automatic thoughts: "Jeremy is the best-looking man at work. He's just perfect, like a Prince Charming. Everything he says and everything he does reminds me of a movie star. I can imagine what it would be like to have his arms around me. Sometimes I feel that if I could just have one kiss, I would die happy." *Voluntary thoughts*: "I've got to remember that he's the best looking man at work *to me*. This is my perception. And it may not be shared by others. And of course he's not perfect. I just think he is because I don't know him that well. So I project my own hopes and wishes on him. The Jeremy I'm mooning over isn't a real person. He is a fictional character, a creation of my own imagination."

Automatic thoughts: "Tricia drives me wild. I'm crazy about her. Those eyes! Those lips! I see her talking to other people and watch how she tosses her head and laughs. And it's as if I'm watching a person in another world, a kind of goddess. If she could be mine I would be the happiest man in the world. *Voluntary thoughts*: "I'm being pretty superficial here. All I'm responding to are Tricia's physical characteristics. I know almost nothing about her personality. I'm inventing the goddess image. She's a creature of flesh and blood just like me. She has her failings and her imperfections. I just don't know what they are. I can't tie my sense of well being to my mind's overactive imaginings."

PROVERBS

Memorize and Mentally Recite Proverbs That Tend to Be Antagonistic to Automatic Thoughts. Certain proverbs are naturally antagonistic to automatic thoughts. These are tried-and-true observations that summarize years of human experience. Think of them as capsules of wisdom. Voluntarily recite one or several appropriate proverbs when you find yourself locked into a self-defeating loop of automatic thoughts that feed into each other.

Here are some examples:

- Into each life a little rain must fall.
- Every cloud has a silver lining.

- Don't cry over spilled milk.
- Every horse thinks its own pack is the heaviest.
- Anger without power is folly.
- Laugh and the world laughs with you. Cry and you cry alone.
- Beauty is in the eye of the beholder.
- Nothing goes right for everybody all of the time.
- Today is the tomorrow we worried about yesterday.
- Life is too serious to take it seriously.

Collect proverbs that are particularly meaningful to you. Then make it a point to say one or several these wise expressions to yourself when you catch sleep-stealing automatic thoughts running through your head.

The Last Word

A counseling client once said to me, "I tried to do what you said. I tried to make my mind go blank. But it didn't work."

Somehow I had been misunderstood. I hadn't advised the individual to make his mind go blank. The literary critic Clifton Fadiman said, "Insomnia is a gross feeder. It will nourish itself on any kind of thinking, including thinking about not thinking." As Fadiman suggests, it is not possible to will yourself to not think. You can't force your mind to go blank.

Consequently, the most practical approach is to employ the strategy of substituting voluntary realistic thoughts for negative automatic ones. This will have a tranquilizing effect. Drowsiness and sleep will then follow in a natural manner.

Key Points to Remember

- Anxiety, anger, guilt, depression, and lovesickness are emotional states that tend to interfere with sleep.

- Emotions have two basic dimensions: (1) an unpleasant-pleasant dimension and (2) a calm-excitement dimension.

- The *cognitive theory* of emotions asserts that it is possible to voluntarily modify our moods to some extent.

- *Automatic thoughts* arise without reflections, are often irrational, and frequently generate negative emotional states.

- *Voluntary thoughts* require an act of will and are well considered. Based on reason and intelligence, they can undercut the adverse effects of automatic thoughts.

- Learn to look upon your worrying as a useless mental activity that generates unnecessary anxiety.

- Take the viewpoint that anger is a form of self-indulgence.

- Realize that much of your guilt may arise from an overly strict superego.

- Put the day's disappointments into a larger perspective.

- Recognize that lovesickness has its origins in idealization.

- Memorize and mentally recite proverbs that tend to be antagonistic to automatic thoughts.

4 THE MEANING OF DREAMS: THE NEED FOR REM SLEEP

Perhaps you are familiar with this quatrain:

In bed we laugh.
In bed we cry.
In bed we're born.
In bed we die.

It might also be added that in bed we dream. Adults spend about 20 percent to 25 percent of the night in rapid eye movement (REM) sleep. Infants spend about 50 percent of their sleeping time in REM episodes.

Why do we dream?

Are dreams necessary for mental health?

Do dreams have meaning?

Can you learn to interpret your own dreams?

Can an understanding of the dreaming process help you get a good night's sleep?

The main body of the chapter will provide general answers to these questions. Toward the end, specific answers will be provided in a brief summary.

Rapid Eye Movement (REM) Sleep

As already indicated, adults spend about 20 percent to 25 percent of their sleeping time in REM sleep. It is impossible to understand sleep without some comprehension of the importance of its REM phases.

As indicated in Chapter 2, REM sleep is associated with light sleep. This kind of sleep obtains its name from the fact that during a REM episode an observer can actually see the eyeballs moving rapidly, seemingly at random, below the eyelids. If an EEG recording is made during REM sleep, the cycles will have a rate of about fourteen per second. The tracings will be "busy" and complex.

Using language with accuracy, we should not say that REM sleep *is* dreaming sleep. Instead, we should say that REM sleep is *associated* with dreaming sleep. The distinction may at first seem trivial, but it is not. If a person is awakened during a REM episode, he or she will usually report a dream. In 80 to 85 percent of such interruptions, a dream is communicated to an observer. However, it is important to realize that in 15 to 20 percent of cases, a dream is *not* communicated.

Conversely, if an individual is awakened during deep sleep, a dream will seldom be reported. However, *sometimes* a dream is reported. If one is reported, its content is usually vague and there is seldom a clearly defined dream story.

These considerations make it evident that a REM episode is a *sign* of dreaming, but not dreaming itself. It is a useful sign in research, but that's all. On the other hand, a dream is an *experience*. Consequently, from your point of view as a subject who is trying to improve the quality of your life, it is what you "see" and "hear" and otherwise sense in a dream that should be of paramount interest. From your dream experiences, you can learn much that is useful, understanding that will in turn help you get a good night's sleep.

The importance of both REM sleep and its association with dreaming will be discussed in this chapter.

What You Can Do

There are a number of things you can do to (1) ensure that you get plenty of REM sleep and (2) derive something of value from your dreams. Although it might appear that both REM sleep and dreaming are involuntary by definition, there are specific actions that will allow you to take partial control of these processes. As you will see, your will and your intelligence have important roles to play.

DRUGS

Avoid Drugs That Inhibit REM Sleep. This point was made in chapter 2, so it will only be referred to briefly here. Sleeping pills are drugs that may inhibit or interfere with REM sleep. So they should be used sparingly, not for chronic behavioral insomnia.

Alcohol is also a drug. It helps to induce sleep, but is sometimes linked to early awakening. If so, valuable REM sleep will be lost in the morning hours.

GETTING UP

Don't Get Up Too Early. Let's say that it's 4:30 in the morning. Your alarm is set for 6:00 A.M. So you're entitled to stay in bed for another hour and a half. You are half asleep and half awake. You're tossing and turning. You're thinking, "Maybe I ought to get up. What's the point of this?" If you in fact stay in bed there's a good chance that you will fall into a light sleep, and you may have one or two more REM episodes before you get up. The dreams you have during these episodes will be of particular importance because they are the ones you are most likely to remember. Don't be bothered by their fantastic or weird quality. As you will see, these can be dreams of substantial value in terms of your overall mental health.

In order to ensure that you don't get up too early, you want to make it easy to either stay asleep or go back to sleep. Consequently, two suggestions bear repeating at this point. First, don't put yourself to sleep with alcohol. This tends to short-circuit morning sleep. Second, make sure that your windows keep out the morning light. Even relatively faint amounts of morning light act as awakening cues. They turn off the pineal gland's secretion of melatonin.

RECORDING DREAMS

Record Your Dreams. It is common to hear someone say, "I guess I have dreams. But I don't remember them." For many of us dreams are experienced at the level of *short-term memory*, a kind of mental waiting room. Short-term memory is sometimes called "working memory." And it is quite common to quickly forget anything in short-term memory. For example, you look up a telephone number. You don't write it down, hold it in short-term memory, dial, and make a connection. Shortly after the call is completed, you don't have the slightest idea what the number is. You know that you did briefly hold the number in memory, but now it is completely gone.

Long-term memory, in contrast to short-term memory, is more or less permanent. Many processes foster long-term memory such as (1) the vividness of an experience, (2) repetition, (3) meaningful associations, and (4) writing down information.

Dreams follow exactly the same kind of memory processing as using a new telephone number. If the dream is not written down as soon as you wake up, most of it will be quickly lost. A steady flow of new sensory inputs will promptly erase all traces of the dream. On the other hand, the simple expedient of writing down as much of the dream as you remember will capture the dream for future inspection and interpretation. Consequently, it is a good idea to have a writing pad or a notebook handy. As soon as you arise make rapid rough notes, capturing as much of the dream's details as possible.

What is the purpose of recording your dreams? Previewing a little, you will see that dreams have a lot to do with the quality of your sleep and your personal adjustment. You record a dream in order to deal with it objectively and realistically.

It is a good idea to keep your dreams in a notebook with dated entries. This is preferable to a collection of random scraps of paper. Such a notebook allows you to study trends in your dreaming, including repeated themes.

EMBELLISHING DREAMS

Embellish Your Dreams. If your dreams are written down, you can go back to them and embellish them. You can add details, supply a missing beginning or a missing ending. You can use your imagination and create a work of fiction. The aim of this authorship is not to produce a commercial product. On the contrary, the story you write is *personal*. It is for your eyes only. Elaborating a dream may seem like an artificial process, but it is not. Elaborations are a product of *your* mind; consequently, if they are written out without too much editing or reflection, they are natural extensions of the dream itself.

Psychiatrist Carl Jung suggested that you nurture the seed of a dream and help it blossom into a fantasy of richer quality. You need not do this only in writing. For example, if you have even a trace of artistic ability, you can try to draw a picture or pictures of what you have seen in the dream. Or you can make a painting of the dream. If you have musical ability, set the dream to music. All of these activities will open doors into the dream and provide you with psychological information of a high quality, information that will make it possible for you to discover the meaning of a dream.

Additional purposes of embellishing a dream will become evident as we proceed.

VOLUNTARY DAYDREAMING

Engage in Voluntary Daydreaming. We all daydream. In most cases daydreams are involuntary fantasies. Daydreams are real dreams. They are produced by the same psychological processes that produce night dreams. Daydreams, like night dreams, are very useful for your mental health. If interpreted properly, they give you insight into the workings of the self. (The art of interpreting dreams will be discussed under the subheading "Interpreting Dreams" later in this chapter.)

You don't have to rely only on involuntary daydreams. You can engage in voluntary daydreaming. One of the principal values of this activity is that such daydreams may be antagonistic to nightmares. If you consciously produce fantastic images, fearful figures, dangerous situations, and so forth, you are less likely to be at the mercy of such psychological content when you are sleeping. They will be less frightening if induced in the light of day.

One way to engage in voluntary daydreaming to is write down the daydream rapidly in response to a stimulus. Below are some examples of stimuli in the form of incomplete sentences. Finish the sentences. And then associate to the completed sentence. Write down whatever comes to mind without regard to logic. If the images are fantastic, like those encountered in a fairy tale, this is desirable. Such images allow the unconscious elements in your mental life an outlet.

1. I am walking down an unfamiliar street. I meet a stranger and . . .

2. Somehow I have been turned into an animal. The animal I have been turned into is . . .

3. I am living in the days of the cave people. There is a famine. The people are dirty and starving and I . . .

4. It is the far future. A few people have attained the power of immortality. I am one of them. My spouse, however is mortal and I . . .

5. I have met the perfect person of the opposite sex. This is my soul mate. He or she embraces me, caresses me, and speaks words of love. We kiss and then . . .

6. I am being given a savage beating. I am bruised and bleeding. But I manage to turn the tables and get the upper hand. Now I have the other person at his or her mercy and . . .

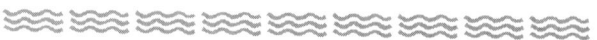

7. I am very old. I am standing nude in front of a full-length mirror. I stare into my own eyes and . . .

Let your imagination run free and write out completions running to a page or two in length. Keep these for reflection and interpretation. They are projections from both the subconscious and unconscious levels of your mind, and they can tell you much about yourself. Also, remember, that this exercise will probably short-circuit any tendency you might possess toward having nightmares.

RESISTING DREAMS

Don't Resist Dreams. Some people resist the dreaming process. They are afraid of their dreams. Dreams confuse, bewilder, and upset them. As a consequence, these same people resist sleeping because this means they will enter the world of dreams. In some cases chronic behavioral insomnia can be an unconscious effort to stay away from the fantastic, threatening universe created by the mind when we dream.

But there is nothing to be afraid of in dreams. They are, after all, only fantasies. They are the mind's attempt to come to grips with the emotional conflicts associated with day-to-day living. And, as already indicated, voluntary daydreaming may reduce the likelihood of having nightmares.

Think of dreams as information. In order to take advantage of this information, you, of course, *do* have to have some way to interpret your dreams. (Again, pointers making this possible are provided later in this chapter under the subheading "Interpreting Dreams.")

AVOIDING NIGHT TERRORS

Avoid Night Terrors by Avoiding Fatigue. Night terrors should not be confused with nightmares. Night terrors are associated with deep sleep, and they are more common in children than adults. A child will abruptly awaken from a deep sleep and be in a state of agitation or mental confusion. Sometimes the child will scream. All the signs of intense fear are present. The child's heart is pounding and there is deep breathing. There is little or no dream content produced by a night terror. With calm reassurance, the child will usually settle down, and often will have no memory of the night terror the next morning.

Although there is no quick and easy way to explain night terrors, they are quite definitely associated with fatigue. A child who is overexcited and goes to bed exhausted is more likely to suffer from night terrors.

What is true of children is also true of adults. An adult prone to night terrors is often a driven person, a compulsive worker, and an individual who generates a high level of self-induced stress. Such a person often goes to bed exhausted at both a physical and an emotional level.

If you suffer from night terrors, examine your general style of life. If you are behaving in such a way as to generate too much fatigue, you may fall into bed in a state of nervous exhaustion. This is the precondition for night terrors. Taking drugs to help you sleep, particularly barbiturates, won't help. On the contrary, they will tend to drive you into deeper sleep and may even aggravate night terrors.

The only practical long-run solution is to reflect on one's work habits and general attitude. Such reflection should make it possible to find ways to avoid excessive fatigue.

For example, Edwin O. is a forty-seven-year-old California real estate broker. He is married and is the father of two children. Here are some remarks he made in a first counseling session. "I'm out for the big bucks. Many evenings I'm on the phone until ten or even eleven. And then I'm studying listing contracts or escrow instructions until midnight. And I've been having night terrors fairly frequently for over five years. They leave me wrung out and I hate them. I've got to find a way to cut them out.

I've tried sleeping pills but they haven't helped. I can't go on this way."

Here are some remarks Edwin made after several counseling sessions. "I haven't had a night terror in three weeks. I've learned to stop working and just do something pleasant and relaxing at least two hours before I go to bed. I'm finding ways to back off a little and not drive myself into a state of nervous exhaustion. I feel better and my general mood has improved."

INTERPRETING DREAMS

Learn to Interpret Your Dreams. If you can learn to interpret your dreams, it will help you acquire a deeper understanding of your own personality. Also, approaching dreams with the confidence of a person who can, to some extent, decipher their meaning, makes you less threatened by them. This in turn helps you overcome resistance to sleep that may arise from a desire to avoid disconcerting dreams.

Three kinds of dreams will be identified and discussed: (1) fantastic dreams; (2) conventional dreams; and (3) numinous dreams.

Fantastic dreams contain elements that make little or no sense in terms of daily life or natural law. Dreams involving objects and events such as flying, giants, magical happenings, living on different worlds, suddenly aging, being a child again, getting trapped in a tunnel, taking a trip in a time machine, living a totally different life than the present one, and so forth suggest the kind of content we are likely to encounter in fantastic dreams.

These were the kind of dreams that were of particular interest to Freud. And they are the most interesting and useful ones in terms of the goal of self-understanding. Freud said that such dreams are "the royal road to the unconscious." In his book *The Interpretation of Dreams*, published almost one hundred years ago, Freud set forth the main keys that enable us to effectively decode fantastic dreams.

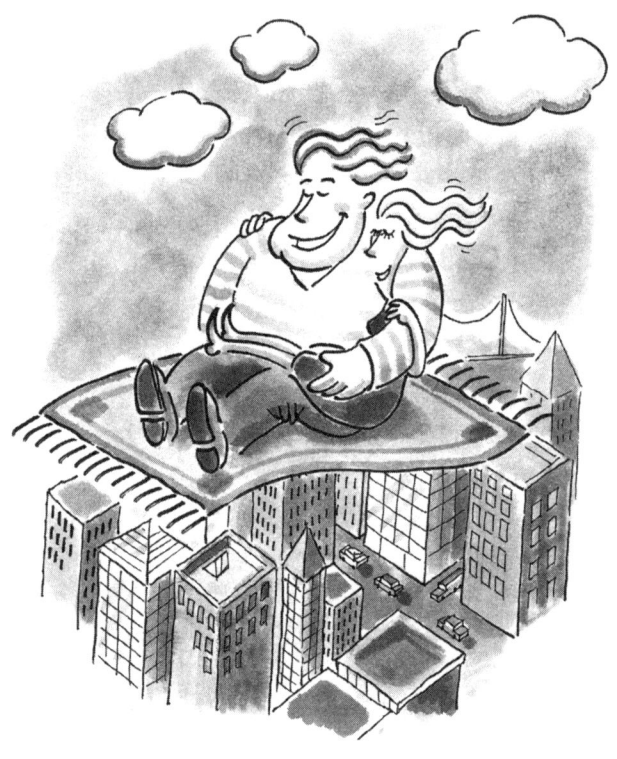

Fantastic dreams have two levels. The first level is called the *manifest level*. It is the surface of the dream. It is the actual dream content—the visualized, heard, or otherwise experienced objects and events of the dream. The dream plot, or story, if there is one, is a part of the manifest content.

The second level is called the *latent level*. It is the hidden side of the dream. It is what the dream means. Freud believed that fantastic dreams are cast in their magical and strange forms in order to conceal the meaning of the dream. The ego, the reality-oriented "I" of the self, steps in and imposes a kind of censorship. This is done in order to maintain self-esteem and avoid feelings of guilt. The manifest content so successfully distorts the latent content that the dream often seems illogical and pointless.

But the dream is *not* illogical and pointless. According to Freud, the latent content usually contains a forbidden wish. This wish is usually of a sexual or aggressive nature. (Remember, at the moment we are talking only about fantastic dreams.)

Arthur C., a thirty-four-year-old attorney, is in business with his father. Arthur dreams that a masked assassin kills a king. When the assassin is caught by the palace guards, instead of being convicted of murder and hung he is magically transformed into the king himself. He steps out on a balcony and the people cheer, "Long live the king! Long live the king!" A wise old sage whispers in his ear, "You will be king forever."

In order to interpret this dream, Arthur can ask himself these kinds of questions:

1. Who does the king stand for in my own life?

2. Who does the masked assassin stand for in my own life?

3. What is the forbidden wish, if any, contained in the dream?

Answers can be obtained by freely associating to the questions. It is useful to put both the questions and their answers in writing.

Arthur's written analysis reveals that the king is his father, the masked assassin is himself, and the forbidden wish is that Arthur's id (defined below) wants to do away with the father and place Arthur in command of the family law firm. This is, of course, a disconcerting interpretation. Does it mean that Arthur wants to kill his father? This is an overly strong statement. Notice that I have been careful to say that Arthur's id wants to do away with the father.

The *id*, according to Freudian theory, is the primitive, fantasy-oriented part of the self. It is totally selfish and cares nothing for reality. But it *is not the whole personality*. Arthur, as a complete person, loves his father. Nonetheless, it certainly can be said that the dream *does* reveal a certain amount of hostility on Arthur's part. He resents his father for being overcontrolling and authoritarian, for running the law firm with an iron hand, and for discounting Arthur's intelligence and contributions to the firm. Looked at in the light of reality, the dream provides a valuable insight into Arthur's relationship with his father.

Kate Y. is twenty-three years old and has been going steady with Jamie for three years. She dreams that Jamie contracts a disease that makes him wither up and age rapidly. As Jamie dies in her arms she sobs and sobs and it seems that her heart is breaking. However, her hair is becoming more luxuriant. Her skin is taking on a lovely glow. Her own health and vitality are being increased by leaps and bounds.

"What a strange dream," Kate thinks. "It shows how much I love Jamie. It must express my fear that my beloved might die."

This is a common-sense interpretation. But if Kate applies the methods described earlier in connection with Arthur, she might look upon the dream in a different light. Instead of expressing a fear for Jamie's life, the dream expresses the precise opposite. The manifest fear is a cover that conceals the forbidden wish. This forbidden wish is, perhaps, not so much that Jamie die, but that he vanish from her life. The dream seems to say that if Jamie were gone, then Kate could have a sort of rebirth of being and spirit. This interpretation will not surprise us if we discover that in waking life Jamie is jealous and possessive and that Kate often feels used and abused by him.

This last point emphasizes the fact that a dream interpretation makes sense only if it fits well with the facts of daily life. A fantastic dream is an expression of real-world concerns, and should be understood in this way.

The events and objects presented at the manifest level of a fantastic dream are *symbols*, meaning they stand for events and objects in the real world. In order to decode a symbol one need only look in the most obvious place: the world of ordinary experience. It is, of course, trite and obvious to say that pens, pencils, guns, bananas, cigars, snakes, and so forth can be symbols of the male phallus. If a genuinely hungry person dreams of eating a banana, then a banana is simply a banana.

Freud was a regular cigar smoker. A hostile colleague once pointed out to Freud that perhaps the cigar was a phallic symbol. Freud's constant sucking and chewing could be a symbol of a forbidden wish to perform an act of fellatio. Unruffled, Freud took the cigar from his mouth, met the other in the eye, and said calmly, "My dear doctor, there are times when a cigar is merely a cigar."

So don't think that the Freudian approach to interpreting your dreams requires you to find all kinds of strange meanings in the symbols you encounter. On the contrary, decode the symbols in terms of your emotional conflicts, your daily frustrations, and your personal goals as a person.

As I have already indicated, it is a good idea to write out questions and answers in connection with the dream. Associating to these will tend to reveal the dream meaning. Take note of the fact also that the strategy presented at the opening of this section recommended that you *learn* to interpret your dreams. Don't expect to interpret your dreams adequately at first. Be patient. Dream interpretation is a trial-and-error process; it is also an uncertain one. It is definitely more of an art than a science. Nonetheless, if you make repeated efforts to interpret your own fantastic dreams, little by little they will give up their meanings to you. And you will obtain those benefits of dream interpretation already specified.

Conventional dreams are straightforward. They are not cast in symbolical form, and, consequently, contain no fantastic element. They are first cousins to fantastic dreams because, like them, they also contain at their core a wish. However, the wish is not a forbidden one.

Therefore the dream does not need to wear a disguise. Symbols are unnecessary.

Phoebe G. is very much in love with Ross. She dreams that it is her wedding day. She sees herself reciting her vows. The wish is transparent. She is impatient to get married and start this new phase of her life.

Rudolph O. is a songwriter. He has had a few songs published, but so far they have enjoyed only modest popularity. He dreams that one of his songs becomes a hit and the money starts rolling in. Again, the wish is transparent. Rudolph wishes to become a successful songwriter, something that he also consciously wishes for in daily life.

A conventional dream is merely an elaborated expression of our natural desires, desires we experience on a regular basis in everyday life. They are good for our mental health in the same way that daydreams are also useful. Conventional dreams allow us to enjoy in fantasy what we may not yet have in reality. They provide an emotional outlet, by granting a wish, for frustrations we may experience in the real world.

You don't have to go to any particular effort to interpret conventional dreams. As indicated, their meanings are more or less self-evident. Only a little reflection is required to see the wish imbedded in the dream.

Numinous dreams evoke feelings of fascination or awe. Awakening from the dream, one has a sense of well being. The dream is well remembered and treasured for a lifetime. These kinds of dreams were of particular interest to the psychiatrist Carl Jung, one of the principal founders of modern psychotherapy. Jung believed that numinous dreams are very special dreams arising not from the level of the personal unconscious, but from the deepest reaches of human nature. Again, a wish or a desire is to be found in the dream. But this time the wish is neither forbidden nor ordinary. The wish is likely to reflect a profound aspect of life and being such as the need for self-actualization or the will to meaning.

The need for *self-actualization* is the need to make the most of your talents and your potentialities. The *will to meaning* is an intense desire to make sense out your life and to discover value in existence.

Priscilla L. reported the following numinous dream in her dream journal. "A white-haired lady is standing on a mountaintop surveying a luxuriant green valley below. The wind is blowing through her hair and she feels triumphant. In spite of the white hair, she is not old. Her face is young and radiant. There is a glorious castlelike structure close at hand. As she approaches it she discerns that its building blocks are books. The castle door opens and she is able to enter it. She quickly learns that she is the queen of the castle."

Priscilla is a thirty-four-year-old divorced woman with young children. Here is a portion of her own commentary on the dream. "I am the woman in the dream. The white hair suggests the passage of time. So the dream is taking place in the future. The young radiant face suggests that even when I am older I will be young at heart. I think that the dream represents my highest aspiration, to become a successful novelist. The dream is one of triumph. Consequently, I am telling myself from the very center of my being that I have the inborn talent to become the person I yearn to be. The dream makes me feel good about myself and reassures me." Clearly, Priscilla's dream is one inspired by the need for self-actualization.

Ralph L. reported the following numinous dream in his journal. "I am on my death bed. It is a big, brass bed and I am surrounded by a loving family. Although I am a widower, my wife is present and alive again in the dream. She is young once more and smiling at me; there is a great radiance emanating from her. My four children and my seven grandchildren are there to say good-bye. But there is no sadness. It is more like the kind of get together that people have on a boat when they want to wish a traveler a bon voyage. I feel very content as they smile at me and I smile back. There is a strong feeling that life has been good and rewarding."

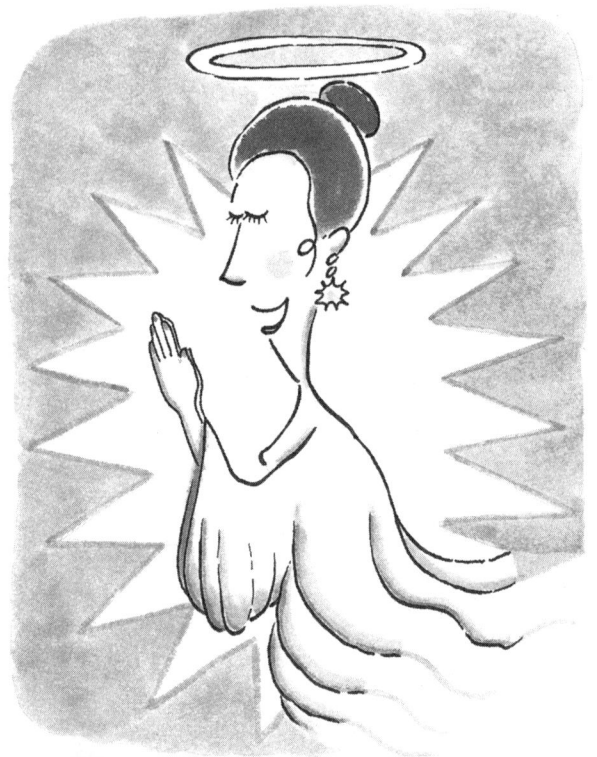

Ralph is over sixty years old. His wife died when she was fifty-four. He was fifty-seven at the time. He is planning to retire soon from a career as a grocery store manager for a supermarket chain. Here is a portion of his own commentary on the dream. "The meaning of this dream is clear. I love my children and my grandchildren. And they love me. They are the lights of my life. I enjoyed raising them. And I took great pleasure in sharing the joys of parenthood with my wife when she was alive. My real vocation in life has been being a parent, not being a store manager. That was a job that I rather liked and was good at. But the really important thing to me has always been my family. The big brass bed shows that I'm important in a way, a kind of VIP to my family." Clearly, Ralph's dream is inspired by the will to meaning. He perceives being a parent as a social role possessing intrinsic value.

Numinous dreams are in fact relatively easy to understand. This is because they do not contain a repressed wish. Consequently, the symbols in such a dream do not hide or disguise anything. On the contrary, they are automatically chosen by the mind's dream processes to *express* meaning.

A numinous dream can, and should, be treasured for a lifetime. It is a gift from, as earlier indicated, the deepest reaches of human nature. Such dreams are not as common as either fantastic or conventional dreams. Consequently, when they spontaneously present themselves they may be thought of as rare psychological diamonds.

Questions and Answers

Let's return to the five questions asked in the introductory paragraphs of this chapter and provide specific answers to them. In most cases, these answers briefly summarize general observations already made. A few additional observations are offered.

Why do we dream? Dreaming appears to serve several purposes. First, there is evidence that dreams help us to classify and reclassify information. It is a process similar to reorganizing files in a filing cabinet. A more contemporary analogy is to say that it is a process similar to reorganizing data on a computer's hard disk. This is a probable explanation of why infants spend 50 percent of their sleeping time in REM sleep. Lacking experience, they have a lot of new data to organize and sort into categories.

Second, in older children and adults dreams express wishes. Some of these wishes are forbidden. And fantastic dreams allow us a unique opportunity to gratify these wishes in fantasy with a minimum of guilt. Although conventional and numinous dreams neither involve forbidden wishes nor guilt feelings, they also function to grant wishes in fantasy form.

Third, dreams preserve sleep. This was a function stressed by Freud. The argument is that a forbidden wish may threaten to break through from the unconscious level of the personality and present itself in raw form. The resulting guilt and anxiety would wake us up. Consequently, the dream process manufactures a symbol to conceal the psychological truth from the dreamer. Anxiety is reduced and sleep is preserved.

Are dreams necessary for mental health? The answer appears to be yes. This seems evident in terms of the functions described in connection with the first question. Safe episodes of controlled psychosis at night can be thought of as an emotional safety valve. It has been said, "We go mad at night so that we can be rational during the day."

Do dreams have meaning? I have met more than one person who believes that dreams are meaningless jumbles of ridiculous images. Even a few psychologists have compared them to the static that one hears on the radio. Static is said to be random "noise" that interferes with "signal." Consequently, it has no informational content. The bulk of evidence seems to be contradictory to this point of view. Research on psychotherapy in particular provides a bounty of evidence suggesting that dreams have meaning. These meanings have already been described in connection with the first question. The key to decoding the meaning of a dream is to realize that in the real world we are often frustrated. Consequently, the meaning of a dream is usually to be found, depending on the kind of dream, in either a concealed wish or a self-evident one.

Can you learn to interpret your own dreams? The answer is yes. But don't expect to skillfully interpret your dreams without experience. The key word here is *learning*. Learning is a trial-and-error process, meaning your skill improves with repetition. Write down your dream.

Include as much detail as possible. Then make associations to the objects and events in the dream. Ideally, keep consecutive dated entries in a binder. Rereading entries will yield additional insights and new associations. Little by little dream meanings will come into focus and become evident to you.

This is not a process of idle curiosity. The meanings you discover in your dreams provide valuable understandings that can help you cope with day-to-day problems.

Can an understanding of the dreaming process help you get a good night's sleep? Again, the answer is yes. If you understand the dreaming process and appreciate its valuable functions, you are less likely to be threatened by the world of dreams. In turn you are less likely to subconsciously resist going to sleep. Put in positive terms, if you become comfortable with the world of dreams, you are likely to look forward to entering that world at night. And, consequently, you will look forward to sleeping because the sleep state is the only gateway we know of into the world of dreams.

The Last Word

Walt Disney and Sigmund Freud are not names that we usually associate with each other. "A Dream Is a Wish Your Heart Makes" is the title of one of the songs in the Walt Disney film *Cinderella*. This song, in a few words, captures the essence of the Freudian theory of dreaming. The word *heart* is used in popular songs as a metaphor to indicate an agent of the personality that is concerned principally with emotions. This is similar to Freud's concept of the id, the primal emotion-oriented self.

As we have seen, a forbidden wish resides at the core of fantastic dreams. And guilt-free wishes play an important part in both conventional and numinous dreams. Consequently, the song's theme that a dream is a wish your heart makes effectively summarizes a most important truth about dreams.

If you would understand your own heart, your own emotional life, look to your dreams.

Key Points to Remember

- Rapid eye movement (REM) sleep is associated with dreaming sleep.
- Avoid drugs that inhibit REM sleep.
- Don't get up too early. Morning dreams during light sleep are often dreams of particular importance.
- Record your dreams. We tend to forget dreams because of the short-term memory process.
- Embellish your dreams.
- Engage in voluntary daydreaming.
- Don't resist dreams.
- Avoid night terrors by avoiding fatigue.
- Learn to interpret your dreams.
- Fantastic dreams have a manifest level and a latent level. The latent level of a fantastic dream is likely to contain a forbidden wish.
- Conventional dreams are straightforward. They express a wish, but not a forbidden one.
- Numinous dreams evoke feelings of fascination or awe. They tend to be well remembered and treasured for a lifetime.
- Dreaming appears to serve several purposes. Among these purposes, Freud proposed that dreams help us to preserve sleep.

5 WHEN LIFE IS DISORGANIZED: FORMING GOOD SLEEP HABITS

Leah H. is a full-time homemaker and the mother of two children. Her daughter is seven and her son is ten. Leah has no particular bedtime, although she insists on a regular one for the children. One night she will go to bed at 10:00 P.M. if she is particularly tired. Another night she will stay up until 3:00 A.M. baking a cake, paying bills, or watching a late, late show. Most mornings she gets up fairly early so that she can help the children get ready for school. Sometimes she sleeps late and her husband, Dexter, sees to it that the children get to school.

Leah suffers from chronic insomnia, and she wonders why. Her physician has assured her that she does not have a physical illness. Dexter, a man who has a defined bedtime as well as a retirement ritual, says, "It's your habits. Or, I should say, your absence of habits. You don't have any. You need to get an organized sleep pattern going. You can't behave just any old way at night."

Dexter is on the right track. Leah's insomnia is behavioral. Her sleep is not induced night after night on a regular basis by predictable cues. And it is difficult to sleep soundly under these circumstances.

Medicine, psychiatry, and psychology employ the term *sleep hygiene* to identify healthy sleep habits. It is worthwhile to establish a set of such habits. They will go a long way to eliminating sleep difficulties.

Approximately twenty-eight hundred years ago the Greek poet Hesiod wrote, "It is best to do things systematically, since we are only human, and disorder is our worst enemy."

If your behavior is anything like Leah's, you can take a lesson from Hesiod's wise observation. Taking a look at your habits, or lack of them, can be of real significance in your search for a good night's sleep. Positive habits promote system and order; and this in turn promotes relaxation and sleep.

Habits

Before we proceed, let's give a little consideration to the concept of habit. A *habit* is a learned response pattern. It is important to place an emphasis on the word *learned*. We are not born with habits. Consequently maladaptive habits can be extinguished ("broken") or modified. And new adaptive habits can be acquired. There is much hope in the concept of habit.

As the concept of habit is used in this chapter, it will refer primarily to regular behavior patterns associated with the preretirement interval, a period of time lasting one to two hours. It is important to organize your time and your life intelligently during this interval. You need, so to speak, a retirement ritual; and this ritual consists of a set of habits. The ritual, if it is the right one for you, will tend to induce sleep.

Although the behaviors that induce sleep will require voluntary effort at first, they will eventually become automatic. When they cross over from the voluntary to the automatic domain, that is when these behaviors become in fact habits. At that point, sleep-inducing habits will become second nature.

Acquiring Sleep-Inducing Habits

Below you will find a group of related behaviors that will, if repeated with a positive intention, become sleep-inducing habits. There is nothing unusual about these behaviors. On the contrary, they are compatible with the way in which your natural circadian rhythm seeks to operate. Therefore, sleep-inducing habits are also habits of health.

BEDTIME

Decide Upon a Regular Bedtime. Everyone is familiar with the concept of a bedtime. In a well-organized family, the children usually have a bedtime. The odds are that you had a bedtime when you were a child.

Adults often depart from the concept of a bedtime. There is the notion of the "night life." In the song "Lullaby of Broadway" from the musical film *Gold Diggers of 1935*, we are told that Manhattan babies don't sleep until the dawn. (Of course, one could say that this *is* their bedtime.) Casinos in cities such as Las Vegas cater to those who seek to gamble well past midnight.

Many of us like Leah have no regular bedtime. We let our transient wishes and momentary desires blow like an emotional wind on the weather vane of time. And we become creatures of impulse as opposed to creatures of habit. As a consequence, our circadian rhythms are totally disrupted and predictable sleep becomes a problem.

What works for actual children will work for the child self that still resides deep within your personality. You must respect this aspect of the self and realize that its requirements still need to be met. It is comforting to have a bedtime. It makes us feel secure. And anything that makes us feel secure helps to promote sleep.

What should be your bedtime? The average adult needs about seven hours of sleep per day. Individual differences suggest that some adults need eight hours; others do well on six hours. You have to make this determination yourself.

Let's say that you have decided that you need about seven hours a day. Let's also say that in terms of your daily schedule you need to arise at 6:00 A.M. Consequently, your bedtime should be between 10:30 and 10:45 P.M.

Why not 11:00 P.M. if you need seven hours? It takes about ten to twenty minutes for most of us to actually fall asleep after we go to bed. So some allowance should be made for this presleep interval.

Perhaps you are offering objections to the idea of a regular bedtime. Here are some common ones:

"What if friends come over to visit and I can't get rid of them until midnight or later?"

"What if we're invited to a party?"

"What if my child is sick and I have to act as a nurse during the night?"

"What if I am the parent of an infant and can't always go to bed when I want to? And, also, what if I have to get up several times during the night to take care of the baby?"

The general answer to the objections is that, of course, there will be times when you can't observe your bedtime. (And there will be times when circumstances won't allow you to stay in bed.) Nonetheless, having a defined bedtime *is* important. You should observe it whenever possible. When you make exceptions, as you will, these will be perceived as disruptions. And you will, if observing a bedtime is a habit, yearn to get back to your normal routine.

In brief, we can say that a regular bedtime acts as a conditioned stimulus. A *conditioned stimulus* is a learned stimulus that triggers an involuntary response. In this case, the response is sleeping. It is very important to have the association even if it is not observed every single day.

GETTING UP

Get Up at a Regular Time. A regular time to climb out of bed was referred to above. Its importance needs to be stressed. For example, if you set an alarm clock for 6:00 A.M., you will frequently find that waking up, like falling asleep, will become a conditioned response. Many of us discover that we automatically wake up a few minutes before the alarm goes off. This is an example of *reverse conditioning*. The response occurs *before* the presentation of the conditioned stimulus.

What is less obvious is that, in terms of your biological clock, there is a gradient of reverse conditioning extending all the way back to your bedtime. What this means in practical terms is that getting up at a regular time also helps you to *fall asleep at a regular time*.

INDUCING RELAXATION

Begin to Induce Relaxation About an Hour Before You Actually Go to Bed. A high level of central nervous system arousal is experienced as alertness and excitement. This is, of course, one of the prime thieves of sleep. If you are "on," you obviously can't be "off." Relaxation is incompatible with high arousal and excitement. Consequently, it is a good idea to make it a point to induce relaxation earlier than the time you plan to retire.

You can't just sit in a chair and say to yourself, "OK, you! Get with it! Relax!" You can't give yourself an order to relax. Relaxation is not under the direct control of the will. However, it is relatively simple to induce relaxation. Below are some easy-to-use induction skills. Think of these as *options*. Use one or several of them at different times in accordance with your own temperament.

Play some soft music. Soft, slow music tends to induce automatic relaxation. Fast, loud music is stimulating and induces excitement. For many persons, instrumental music alone is more relaxing than a vocal backed up by music.

Dim the lights. Light, as already noted, has been called a "gatekeeper" for sleep. Light helps the pineal gland *generate* melatonin. But the generation and storage of melatonin is not the same as secretion. Light inhibits the *secretion* of melatonin. And this is required for you to fall asleep. You can get a head start on the process of secretion by dimming lights and reducing overall illumination about an hour before you go to bed.

Read something familiar or predictable. If reading makes you drowsy, by all means read for about an hour before you retire. For some people the eye fatigue tends to induce sleepiness. However, be sure that what you read is perceived as relatively boring. Consequently, you *don't* want to read a novel with an interesting plot or a thriller. And you certainly *don't* want to read a horror story. No, the safest bet at night is nonfiction. Of course you don't want to read something that is *completely* boring, or why bother to read at all? But if the article or book is something that you can set down readily, if you don't *have to* keep reading, so much the better.

Take a warm bath. Warm water automatically relaxes muscles. Muscle relaxation is antagonistic to anxiety and high arousal. If you take a warm bath about an hour before you retire, you will find yourself automatically letting go and settling down.

Engage in moderate exercise. Moderate exercise about two hours before you go to bed can help you relax. True, exercise in and of itself increases arousal. But shortly after you exercise there is a mild boomerang effect and you will find your body relaxing without an act of will or other effort on your part. Take note of the fact that the word *moderate* has been used. Examples of moderate exercise include going for a short walk, using an exercise bicycle, using a treadmill, doing a few sit-ups, lifting some light weights, and playing a game of Ping-Pong. Fifteen to twenty minutes of activity is enough. And if you are huffing and puffing you are overdoing it. The purpose of this kind of exercise is not to engage in an aerobic session, but to introduce a precondition to relaxation.

EATING AND SLEEP

Have a Light Snack About an Hour Before Retiring. Eating is another way to induce relaxation. I am discussing it under a separate heading because it is a significant subject in itself with several important aspects.

Food is a natural tranquilizer. This is because it stimulates the activity of the parasympathetic division of the autonomic nervous system. The *autonomic nervous system* controls involuntary functions such as digestion, respiration, and pulse. Its *sympathetic division* is a kind of "Go!" system and has the effect of increasing arousal and alertness. The *parasympathetic division* is a kind of "Slow down!" system and has the effect of decreasing arousal and alertness. Eating switches on this system and relaxes you.

However, it is important that the snack you eat be *light*. If too much food is consumed just before retiring, you may experience gastrointestinal distress in bed, and this, of course, will be likely to keep you awake. Specific examples of such distress include flatulence, bloat, and heartburn.

Examples of light snacks that will not tend to produce gastrointestinal distress in most persons include:

A glass of low-fat or nonfat milk

A piece of toast with just a touch of margarine

A piece of fresh fruit

One-half cup of cooked vegetables

Two graham crackers

One-half of a baked potato with just a touch of margarine or olive oil

A raw green pepper

One-half cup of puffed rice

A cup of chicken noodle soup

A slice of low-fat cheese

A slice of turkey

(Note: If you are lactose intolerant, you will want to obtain either lactose-reduced or lactose-free milk and cheese. Some persons find that foods containing lactose create gastrointestinal distress such as cramps and gas.)

The above snacks all contain less than 100 calories. The general principal is to keep the snack high in protein or high in complex carbohydrates. Also, keep the snack low in fat and refined carbohydrates. Snacks such as those recommended are also likely to facilitate serotonin production, a neurotransmitter that helps you sleep. (This was discussed in chapter 2.)

LAUGHTER

Think of Laughter as a Tranquilizer with No Side Effects. Watching a comedian deliver a monologue on television is likely to put you in a good mood. Ideally, this should take place about an hour before you retire. Assuming you are pleasantly amused, not semihysterical with laughter, you will be only slightly excited by what you have watched. When you turn off the television set, the natural counteraction sets in; arousal is automatically lowered. And the kind of relaxation that precedes sleep sets in.

SHIFT WORK

If Possible, Avoid the Frequent Rotation of Shifts. If you work a regular night shift, all that has been said so far still applies. The word *bedtime* does not necessarily imply nighttime. It means "a regular time to retire to bed." So if you work either a late evening shift or a night shift, you should still try to organize your time and your life in such a way that you observe a regular bedtime.

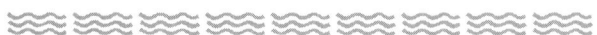

The real problem arises if you frequently rotate shifts. When I worked in the psychiatric unit of a military hospital in the air force the staff observed three shifts: (1) 7:00 A.M. to 3:00 P.M., (2) 3:00 P.M. to 11:00 P.M., and (3) 11:00 P.M. to 7:00 A.M. Also, the unit had to be covered on weekends and holidays. Under these conditions, most of us who worked on the unit, when given the option, selected one shift for a prolonged period of time (three months, for example). This gave us the opportunity to settle down to a routine, a bedtime, and a predictable sleep pattern.

When we went from one shift to another, we had to make adjustments. Our circadian rhythms were disrupted. Our biological clocks had to be reset. It is usually said that in order to overcome jet lag it requires about one day of adjustment for each hour of time zone crossed. A similar rule applies to shift work. If the lag period is eight hours or more, as it is when you switch from sleeping in the day to the night or vice versa, then the adjustment period required is about a week. If it takes you this long to readjust, don't get angry with yourself or think that something is wrong with you. You are on a normal readjustment timetable and nature is taking its course.

The really important thing to do in terms of shift work is, as indicated above, to restrict the frequency of the rotations. Sticking with one shift for about three months, if you can, is optimal. This means you will only have to readjust your biological clock four times a year, which is quite enough for anyone.

LATE-NIGHT SEX

Engage in Late-Night Sex Only If You Are Relatively Confident That You Will Have an Orgasm. We are told in songs and poems that "the night was made for love." Some experts even recommend late-night sex as a way to relax. And this is good advice if you are relatively confident that you will have an orgasm. Immediately following an orgasm your body automatically goes into a state of low arousal, a state that facilitates falling asleep. However, this seemingly simple process frequently goes haywire.

Let's review the four stages of the sexual response cycle. These are (1) excitement; (2) plateau; (3) orgasm; and (4) resolution. Let's take a familiar measure of arousal such as pulse rate. Let us say that before sexual excitement your resting pulse is 70 beats per second. You are in a state of normal arousal.

During Stage 1, or *excitement*, assume that with sexual stimulation your pulse rate rises to 90 or 100 beats per minute. During Stage 2, or *plateau*, your pulse rate remains at 90 or 100 beats per minute. The plateau phase can last from two to twenty minutes depending on various factors.

During Stage 3, or *orgasm*, the pulse rate may briefly shoot up to 120 beats per minute or higher. Orgasm is both a physiological event and a psychological experience. At the physiological level, the female has involuntary contractions of the *pubococcygeus (PC) muscle*, a muscle surrounding the vaginal channel. In the male, bladder muscles contract and *compressor muscles* around the urethra relax. And there is an ejaculation of semen. In both sexes, at a psychological level, the orgasm is experienced as the peak of sexual pleasure.

During Stage 4, or *resolution*, the pulse rate usually drops down below the original resting pulse. Deep relaxation is induced and sleep often follows relatively soon and easily.

However, both males and females can suffer from *sexual dysfunction* including inhibited orgasm, male erectile dysfunction, and painful intercourse. Males are quite a bit more likely to enjoy an orgasm as a result of intercourse than are females. There are various reasons for this. The male may ejaculate before the female has an orgasm. It is then next to impossible to continue penile stroking. If the male is unwilling to provide other stimulation, or if the female finds it offensive to engage in autostimulation, she

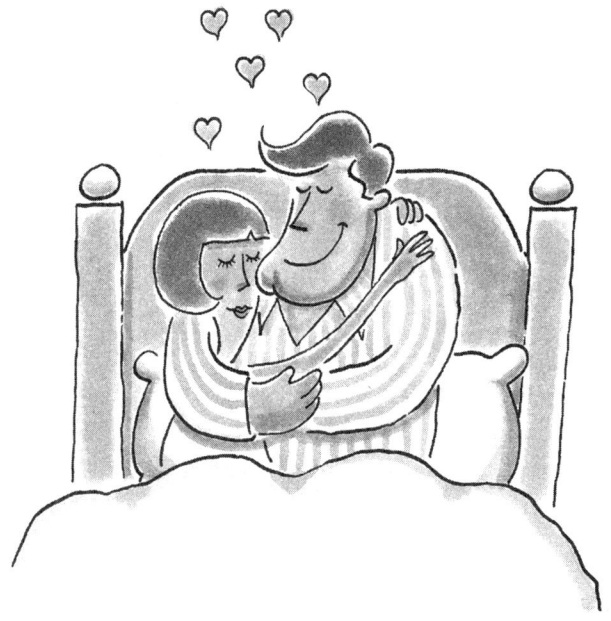

will remain in Stage 2, excitement, for a prolonged period. Or the female may suffer from a specific kind of sexual dysfunction called *inhibited orgasm* (also called *orgasmic dysfunction*). She will become excited, but will have difficulty reaching a climax. Again, she will remain in an excited state with no quick and easy resolution. Obviously, a sexually excited person who feels frustrated and deprived of an orgasm has a difficult time falling asleep.

If you suffer from a sexual dysfunction, you and your partner are, of course, encouraged to seek solutions. Possibly you will want to see a therapist. In any event, you *don't* want to try to work out your sexual problems immediately before seeking a good night's sleep. The two objectives are clearly contradictory.

SLEEP AND PRAYER

If It Is Compatible with Your World View, by All Means Say a Bedtime Prayer. Many persons, even those who believe in the effectiveness of prayer, have gotten away from the habit of saying a bedtime prayer. Such a prayer can have a very calming effect and help you to go to sleep.

Rebecca H., a forty-seven-year-old insurance broker, wife, and mother, says, "I say the Lord's Prayer every night before I go to sleep. I say it in bed with my eyes closed. After I finish the prayer I ask God to bless my family and the people I love. I think about the whole human race, and I always conclude my prayer with a line from Charles Dickens's *A Christmas Carol*. That line is, 'God bless us one and all.' My prayer really helps me to fall asleep."

Carson L., a fifty-two-year-old army general, husband, and father, says, "I find it particularly comforting to recite the Twenty-third Psalm before I go to bed. It's the one that begins, 'The Lord is my shepherd. I shall not want.' There is no doubt to me that it is one of the most comforting of the psalms."

You do not, of course, have to recite prewritten prayers. You can pray in your own way in your own words. In Richard Llewellyn's novel *How Green Was My Valley*, the minister Mr. Gruffydd tells the book's narrator, a boy named Huw:

> *Prayer is only another name for good, clean, direct thinking. When you pray, think well what you are saying, and make your thoughts into things that are solid. In that manner, your prayer will have strength, and that strength shall become part of you, mind, body and spirit.*

A RITUAL

Have a Retirement Ritual. A retirement ritual consists of a predictable sequence of bedtime habits. The ritual should be started about an hour before you go to bed. Each habit in the ritual helps you to relax and prepares your mind and body to fall asleep. Go back over the suggestions in this chapter. Select three or four that have particular appeal to you. Adapt them to you own individual needs, and make them a part of your ritual.

Harrison L., a forty-year-old insurance agent, says, "Every night about an hour before I go to bed I put on my robe. This gives me a cozy feeling. I make myself a cup of decaffeinated coffee and put in a generous amount of nonfat milk. I have it with a slice of whole grain toast with a half-teaspoon of peanut butter spread on it.

"I sit in my favorite chair, a big one in the family room. I read. But I make it a point to avoid reading anything about the insurance business. I use a lamp that casts an indirect light, bouncing back from the ceiling. There's no glare on the page that way. The overall illumination is low.

"My wife, Vanessa, and I sometimes have the television set on. But we seldom watch the late news. We usually watch one or two news shows earlier in the evening. The late news gets me upset and can interfere with my sleep. Vanessa has her own routine that includes, as mine does, putting on her robe about an hour before we go to bed."

The Last Word

Imagine that you are driving a car. You are traveling at the rate of sixty miles per hour. There is a stop sign up ahead.

Do you wait until the last minute to use your brakes? Or do you begin to slow down before you arrive at the stop sign? The answers are obvious. An experienced driver *prepares* to stop.

Going to sleep follows the same logic as that used when we drive. It is a good idea to slow down and *prepare* yourself for the cessation of normal consciousness associated with sleep. Slowing down reduces central nervous system arousal and creates a precondition for sleep. If you follow the natural sleep-inducing habits identified in this chapter, you will find them potent agents in your efforts to defeat insomnia.

Key Points to Remember

- Medicine, psychiatry, and psychology employ the term *sleep hygiene* to identify healthy sleep habits.
- A *habit* is a learned response pattern.
- Decide upon a regular bedtime.
- Get up at a regular time.
- Begin to induce relaxation about an hour before you actually go to bed.
- Here are some relatively easy-to-use skills that will induce relaxation: (1) Play some soft music; (2) dim the lights; (3) read something familiar or predictable; (4) take a warm bath; and (5) engage in moderate exercise.
- Have a light snack about an hour before retiring.
- Think of laughter as a tranquilizer with no side effects.
- If possible, avoid the frequent rotation of shifts.

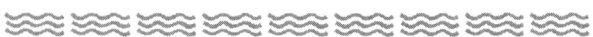

- Engage in late-night sex only if you are relatively confident that you will have an orgasm.
- If it is compatible with your world view, by all means say a bedtime prayer.
- Have a retirement ritual.

6 SELF-HYPNOSIS: A PRACTICAL SLEEP-INDUCTION SKILL

The word *hypnosis* tends to evoke mixed emotional reactions in many of us. On the one hand, we are fascinated by its possibilities. On the other hand, we are somewhat put off by its association with mystical lore.

Hypnosis suffered a big blow to its reputation when it was used to produce so-called miraculous cures by a French charlatan named Franz Anton Mesmer. A committee of scientists was assembled to investigate his extravagant claims. Its members included the U.S. ambassador to France, Benjamin Franklin. The committee concluded that Mesmer's "cures" were frauds. The events described took place about two hundred years ago. To this day another word for hypnosis is *mesmerism*.

Hypnosis has had a checkered history since the days of Mesmer. Freud used hypnosis for a time in psychotherapy with neurotic patients, but gave it up. He decided that the cures it seemed to produce were temporary.

The advantages and disadvantages of hypnosis have been explored from every conceivable angle by both the psychiatric and the psychological professions. The present status of hypnosis is that it has a legitimate place in the effective treatment of certain disorders. The Council on Mental Health of the American Medical Association made a favorable report on hypnosis in 1958. The American Psychiatric Association issued a policy statement in 1961 affirming the use of hypnosis in psychotherapy. Hypnosis has become respectable.

The term *hypnosis* was coined by an Englishman named James Braid. He derived the term from *Hypnos*, the ancient Greek god of sleep. Braid thought of hypnosis as a specific kind of sleep state. This is now believed to be incorrect. Hypnosis is *not* sleep. It is an altered state of consciousness that has a superficial resemblance to sleep. During a hypnotic state, one is somewhat more suggestible than when one is in a normal waking state.

There is, of course, a link between hypnosis and sleep. The heightened suggestibility associated with hypnosis can be used to induce relaxation and sleep. It is this link that we will exploit in this chapter.

Using Self-Hypnosis

It is, of course, possible to seek the services of a professional hypnotist to treat chronic behavioral insomnia. If you decide to do this, check out the individual's credentials carefully. You may be told that the therapist is "licensed." Don't be set at ease too quickly. The license referred to may be a business license, easily obtained with no qualifications. Make sure that the professional person is licensed to practice psychotherapy by a state board of examiners. In most cases, a qualified therapist will be either a psychiatrist or a clinical psychologist.

You can also learn to practice the art of self-hypnosis. There is nothing mysterious or unusual about this. Self-hypnosis takes advantage of the fact that we are sensitive to our own autosuggestions. *Autosuggestions* are statements that we tell ourselves, positive or negative, that tend to have a profound influence on our mental and emotional states, as well as our actions. We engage in this process automatically many times a day. Using self-hypnosis, the autosuggestions are simply somewhat more effective.

Self-hypnosis and autosuggestion can be readily combined to induce sleep.

TRANCE INDUCTION

Learn How to Induce a Self-Hypnotic Trance. The self-induction of a hypnotic trance is not a difficult thing to learn. It is actually a natural process, and, consequently, is something that you can teach yourself to do. You will find a set of step-by-step instructions below. In subsequent sections, additional options and possibilities are offered.

Step 1. Assume that you are reclining in bed and all of the lights are off. If you are on your back, stare up in the dark toward the ceiling. If you are on your side, stare toward the wall or the window.

Step 2. Mentally say to yourself, as if a hypnotist is speaking in your mind, "Imagine a spot of light floating near the ceiling (or the wall or window)."

(Take note of two key points. First, as indicated, it is useful to "hear" the instructions *as if* a hypnotist is speaking to you. Use your creative imagination and perceive the hypnotist's voice as confident and authoritative. Perhaps it is just a shade lower in pitch than your own normal speaking voice. The voice speaks slowly, calmly, and reassuringly. Second, it is not essential to memorize the following script word for word. If you paraphrase and capture the gist of the suggestions, this will be sufficient and effective.)

Now say to yourself, "I am going to count slowly to ten. Keep your eyes open and continue staring at the imaginary spot of light as I count. With each count you will get sleepier and sleepier. When I reach the count of ten you will close your eyes and drift off into a gentle restful sleep lasting until the time that you want to wake up." (The "I" is the imaginary hypnotist; the "you" is you, the subject.)

Step 3. Say to yourself, "One. Keep staring at the light. You are getting a little drowsy. Your eyelids are getting heavy. You feel like yawning. Go ahead and yawn when you decide to."

Step 4. Say to yourself, "Two. Keep looking at the light. You are getting drowsy. Drowsier and drowsier. Your eyelids are getting heavier and heavier. You are letting go of the concerns of the day and relaxing."

Step 5. Say to yourself, "Three. Keep looking at the light. You are getting sleepy. Sleepier and sleepier. So sleepy. It's a good feeling. You are letting go of tension and relaxing . . . relaxing."

Step 6. Say to yourself, "Four. The light is still there—still on. Keep looking straight at it. You are getting drowsier and drowsier. Your eyelids are getting heavier and heavier. Heavier and heavier. You are getting so very, very relaxed."

Step 7. Say to yourself, "Five. The light is there. Keep looking at it. You are getting more and more sleepy. So sleepy. Your eyelids are getting heavier and heavier. You would love to close them. Soon you will be able to do so. Relaxation is spreading throughout your muscles and your very being."

Step 8. Say to yourself, "Six. The light is there. Things are getting fuzzy around it. It's a very pleasant, relaxing sight. You are getting really sleepy now. It would be so good to be able to let go and drift off to sleep. Your eyelids are getting so heavy, so very heavy."

Step 9. Say to yourself, "Seven. You are looking at the light. It seems to be floating in a hazy cloud. You are getting sleepier and sleepier and sleepier. Oh, how much you want to be allowed to let go and begin sleeping. But not yet. Not just yet. Your eyelids are getting heavier and heavier. You want to blink them. Go ahead and blink them."

Step 10. Say to yourself, "Eight. Almost there. Almost there. Still looking at the light. It's floating in a cloud. You are so sleepy . . . so sleepy . . . so sleepy. Your eyelids are so heavy you can barely keep them open."

Step 11. Say to yourself, "Nine. Almost there. Almost there. Still looking at the light. It's growing dim and almost covered by the cloud. You are very, very sleepy. You are very, very sleepy. So sleepy. So sleepy. Your eyelids want to close. They are so very heavy. You are feeling very relaxed and ready to fall asleep."

Step 12. Say to yourself, "Ten. Close your eyes. Soon you will drift into a gentle, refreshing sleep. If you briefly awaken during the night in order use the bathroom, you will be able to go, return to bed, and get back to sleep readily. You will sleep easily until the time you want to wake up."

REVISIONS

Feel Free to Revise and Adapt the Basic Trance Induction Instructions. You now have the basic instructions. If you want to vary them or modify them, in terms of your own personality or your own unique needs, this is a good idea. Be creative and use your own character as a guide. Tell yourself what you need to hear, what will be useful to you. Working from the basic instructions, write out your own script.

AN AUDIOTAPE

It Can Be Useful to Make an Audiotape of the Trance Instructions. If you find it difficult to concentrate and give yourself mental instructions, you can vary the self-hypnotic approach by making an audiotape recording of either the basic script or the one you have written. Vary your own voice slightly. As suggested in connection with the imaginary voice, give your voice a slight air of authority. Speak at a somewhat lower pitch. Use a calm and reassuring tone.

Play the recording when you retire for the evening. If you live alone, or if you have a partner who does not object, then playing the audiotape can be a practical method of self-hypnosis. It will not disturb the trance state if you reach out and push the "off" button on the tape recorder at the conclusion of the instructions.

If you listen to the tape several times, you are likely to find that you can eventually recite the instructions at a

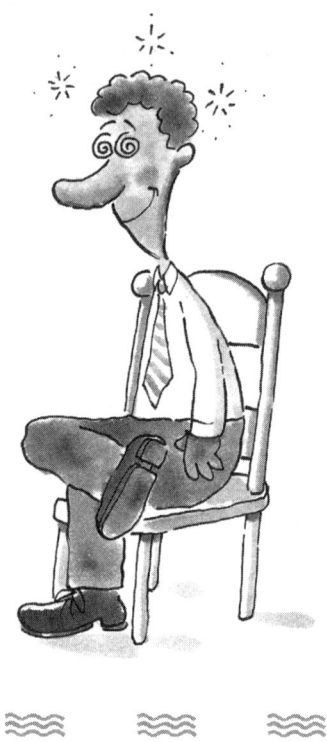

mental level without the aid of a machine. You, in a sense, carry the "tape" with you in your mind.

THE TRANCE STATE

Don't Be Put Off by the Concept of a Trance. The word *trance*, for some persons, smacks of mysticism and the occult. Actually, a trance, as it is being used here in connection with hypnosis can be defined as follows: an altered state of consciousness in which the mind is somewhat more receptive to suggestions. In view of the fact that the suggestions in question are *autosuggestions*, suggestions that you give yourself, there is nothing to fear. You are in complete control of both the trance state and the suggestions. You are giving up neither your will nor your intelligence. On the contrary, you are *using* your will and your intelligence to achieve a practical goal, the goal of creating a psychological frame of reference conducive to a good night's sleep.

AN ACTUAL LIGHT SOURCE

Use an Actual Light Source as a Focusing Device. You may find it difficult to imagine a spot of light. If you prefer, or if it is convenient, you can, of course, use an actual spot of light instead. Many electronic clocks have displays, or partial displays, that stay on all night. Often these contain one or several dots of softly glowing light. Place the clock at a comfortable distance, and stare at the spot of light as you give yourself autosuggestions.

An alternative way to create a spot of light is to place a flashlight in a shoe box. Punch a hole about one-quarter inch in diameter in the shoe box.

You will find that as you stare at it the spot of light seems to be moving. Frequently it jerks around a bit. This is a normal perceptual phenomenon, so don't be disturbed by the experience. It is called the *autokinetic phenomenon*, meaning, roughly, the "self-moving phenomenon." The cause of the autokinetic phenomenon is a physiological process called *involuntary nystagmus*, suggesting that without conscious control your eyeballs move about slightly and at random. This process, not usually noticed, is going on all of the time. Its purpose is to present rested photoreceptors (neurons sensitive to light) in the retina at all times to incoming stimulation.

Another phenomenon associated with staring at an actual spot of light is a *perceptual penumbra*. This is experienced as a cloudy fringe around the spot of light. The perception arises from the fact that when the eye is forced to fixate on a visual target, photoreceptors in the periphery of the retina adapt to light and go into a "dim" mode. (The involuntary nystagmus referred to above is antagonistic to this action; but when you will yourself to fixate on a visual target the nystagmus is not sufficient to completely overcome the adaptation effect.) The penumbra helps you to fall asleep because it helps to create the psychological impression that you are inducing an altered state of consciousness.

GOING BACK TO SLEEP

Use Self-Hypnosis as a Way of Going Back to Sleep. You may not find it difficult to fall asleep when you go to bed. A common pattern associated with behavioral insomnia is to wake up after three or four hours of sleep and find it difficult to go back to sleep. It is 2:00 or 3:00 A.M. and you seem to be wide awake. I say "seem to be" because to some extent your wide-awake condition is an illusion. The odds are that you are still in need of sleep and can fall asleep again fairly readily under the right conditions.

Under the above circumstances, self-hypnosis can be of particular value. Let's say that you have just returned to bed from the bathroom. Recline in a comfortable position, stare at a real or imaginary light, and mentally recite the trance instructions.

Or, if you feel overly restless in bed, get up. There is no rule that says you have to spend all of your sleeping time in bed. Go into a different room and make yourself comfortable in an easy chair, a recliner, or a sofa. Often there will be a tiny light source. The clock on a VCR is convenient for this purpose. Get comfortable, and mentally recite the trance instructions.

A variation on the above strategy is to first have a cup of warm beverage such as decaffeinated coffee or caffeine-free herbal tea, and read for about fifteen minutes. Be sure that the reading light is both indirect and not too bright. Too much light exposure will inhibit the secretion of melatonin. Reading can be useful because in the wee hours of the morning it tends to induce eye fatigue. Tell yourself before you start that you will definitely stop reading when fifteen minutes are up. Look at a clock and determine a time to quit. When the time is up, go to the chair, recliner, or sofa and follow the trance instructions.

REPETITION AND SYSTEMATIC AUTOSUGGESTION

The Twin Keys to Effective Self-Hypnosis Are Repetition and Systematic Autosuggestion. You will note that to some extent the trance instructions are "boring." This is because they involve repetition. In order for autosuggestions to have an impact on the subconscious mind they must be repeated, repeated, and repeated.

Also, there must by *systematic autosuggestion*. This means that the suggestions you give yourself must be given in an orderly, logical, noncontradictory fashion. They must make sense to your conscious mind if they are to make sense to your subconscious mind. Combine these two keys whenever you employ self-hypnosis.

REVERSING SUGGESTIONS

Reverse the Trance Suggestions to Help You Wake Up. In the same way that autosuggestions can help you go to sleep, they can be used to help you become more alert. Let's say that you have just awakened. You feel a little drowsy and your body seems sluggish. Remain in bed with your eyes closed and mentally recite the following:

"I am going to count backward fairly rapidly from seven to one. With each count you will feel more alert and more functional.

"Seven. You are waking up and feeling alert. Stretch. That feels good.

"Six. You are waking up and feeling more and more alert. You feel refreshed and ready to take on the day.

"Five. You are feeling more alert. You feel ready to get up and get going.

"Four. You are feeling more alert and awake. You're ready to get going.

"Three. You are more alert and awake. Your mind is clear. You are refreshed.

"Two. You are alert and awake. Your mind is clear and lucid. You are refreshed. You want to get up and get going.

"One. Open your eyes. You are alert and refreshed. You're ready to get up and get going. Go ahead and get up."

Notice that when using self-hypnosis to wake up the number of suggestions are both fewer and briefer. You can go through this process fairly rapidly. And you don't need a real or imaginary spot of light. The idea is to come out of the sleep state and to enter normal waking consciousness. Just give yourself the autosuggestions in an easy, brisk manner with your eyes closed.

Observe also that the counting is done backward. You went *into* the sleep state by counting forward. Counting backward when coming *out of* the sleep state is useful because it contains the implicit suggestion that you are reversing the original trance suggestions in order to obtain alertness and optimal arousal.

LEARNING

Hypnosis Is a Phenomenon of Learning. More than one study has shown that hypnosis belongs to the learning process. Actually, it may be thought of as a form of conditioning in which the autosuggestions act as *conditioned stimuli*, stimuli to which there are learned responses. The trance and the sleep state induced are *conditioned responses*, semiautomatic responses that are acquired by learning.

Because hypnosis is a phenomenon of learning, it may take a number of repetitions of the trance instructions before you become adept. If you don't get impressive results the first time you try, don't give up. If you go through the basic trance-induction steps outlined earlier, you will find that each time they are repeated a proficiency will develop. Little by little conditioning will set in, and you will find it relatively easy to invoke a sleep-inducing trance.

The Last Word

If you are a skeptic and believe that self-hypnosis is just a lot of bunk, then you will find that it *is*! This is simply because for self-hypnosis to be effective an open mind is required. Autosuggestions have little or no effect on the mental life of a person who is hostile and resistant.

On the other hand, if you have a positive attitude and believe that self-hypnosis can help you to sleep, you will find that it *can*! Predicting that self-hypnosis will help a person sleep falls into the category of a self-fulfilling prophecy. It can help you if you think it can.

So approach self-hypnosis with an open mind. Think in terms of trial-and-error learning. Expect to get good results in the long run.

Key Points to Remember

- The present status of hypnosis is that it has a legitimate place in the effective treatment of certain disorders.

- The term *hypnosis* was coined by an Englishman named James Braid. He derived the term from *Hypnos*, the ancient Greek god of sleep.

- *Autosuggestions* are statements that we tell ourselves, positive or negative, that tend to have a profound influence on our mental and emotional states, as well as our actions.

- Learn how to induce a self-hypnotic trance. The chapter includes step-by-step instructions.

- Feel free to revise and adapt the basic trance instructions.
- It can be useful to make an audiotape of the trance instructions.
- Don't be put off by the concept of a trance.
- If you prefer, or if it is convenient, use an actual light source as a focusing device instead of imagining a spot of light.
- Use self-hypnosis as a way of going back to sleep.
- Understand that the twin keys to effective self-hypnosis are repetition and systematic autosuggestion.
- Reverse the trance suggestions to help you wake up.
- Be aware that hypnosis is a phenomenon of learning.

7 MORE WAYS TO OBTAIN BETTER SLEEP: A CATALOG OF TIPS AND TECHNIQUES

There are many ways to cope with behavioral insomnia. What works for one person will not work for another. Individual differences reign supreme in the world of sleep and dreams.

Sometimes even a single suggestion can make an enormous difference. The critical thing is to find, and apply, the right suggestion for you—one that works in terms of your needs, your situation, and your personality.

Think of this chapter as providing a catalog of sleep-inducing tips and techniques that work for many people. A number of them will almost certainly be helpful to you. The information in this chapter augments and supplements the information provided in prior chapters.

The Catalog

For convenient reference, the suggestions in this "catalog" have been arranged in alphabetical order. Pick and choose from the tips and techniques as you see fit. Take a trial-and-error approach, testing the ideas in your own way. Also, adapt the ideas to your own personality.

ALLERGENS

Provide Yourself with an Allergen-Free Environment. An *allergen* is a substance that is an irritant. The adverse reaction to an allergen is called an allergy. What is an allergen for you may not be an allergen for me. Common allergens include house dust, bird feathers, cat fur, perfumes and colognes, deodorizers, and the airborne pollen from plants. Most parents are aware of the need to provide an allergen-free environment for children. However, they forget that adults have allergic reactions too.

If you are having trouble sleeping, one factor can be allergens in your environment. You may have an adverse reaction to a substance and be only half aware of it. The adverse reaction can cause sneezing, wheezing, fatigue, and headaches. Many of the problems are caused by airborne substances. Clear your environment of the agents that you suspect of producing these substances. For example, Drew W. was allergic to roses. They bothered him if they were anywhere in the house because their pollen was carried through the air ducts.

If it seems virtually impossible to clear your home of all allergens, consider equipping your home with an electronic air filter. This can be made a part of the air-conditioning system. There are also free-standing electronic filters available. Another alternative is to use a cool-water humidifier. This helps to clear the air of microscopic allergens.

It is important to stress that some people have subtle allergic reactions and may not think of themselves as having a problem. Of course one can overreact and have a hypochondriacal reaction, imagining that all sorts of things are allergens that are not. On the other hand, it is a different kind of foolish behavior to ignore the possibility that allergic reactions may be disturbing the quality of one's sleep.

CLOCKS

Remove a Constantly Illuminated Clock from Your Immediate Visual Environment. You are probably familiar with the saying, "A watched pot won't boil." I often

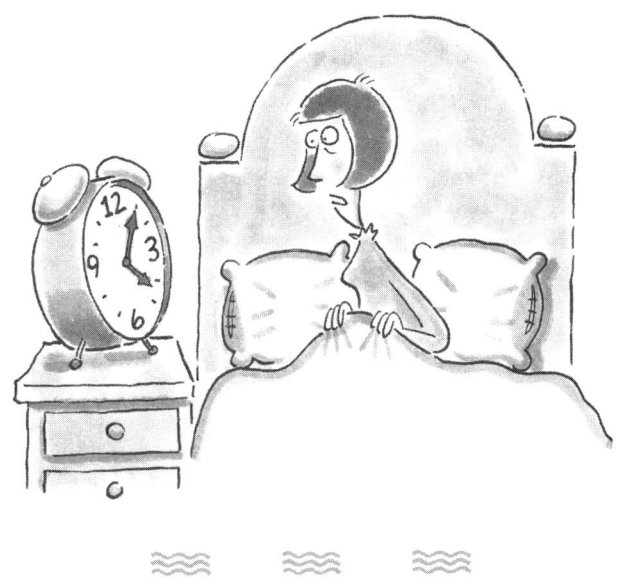

prepare a mug of water for instant coffee by putting it the microwave oven and setting the timer for two minutes. If I stand around in the kitchen waiting for the two minutes to pass, it seems a lot longer than two minutes. If we focus our attention directly on time itself, time seems to pass more slowly, often *too slowly*.

Many electric clocks have constantly illuminated faces. Aside from the fact that the unnecessary light may slightly inhibit the secretion of melatonin, the too-readily available chronological information tends to encourage an excessively high level of *self-monitoring behavior*, behavior in which you reflect on your own behavior and become too aware of it. In this particular instance, during the presleep interval, you look from time to time at the clock face and say to yourself, "Oh, has only three more minutes gone by? It seems like forever!" This kind of perception and thought tends to greatly aggravate restlessness. Soon you will throw back the covers and get out of bed because it seems that it is taking "forever" to go to sleep.

If you have set the clock's alarm, and need it for that purpose, turn the clock's face away from you. Don't be able to look at it without making the slightest effort. If, during the night, you want to find out what time it is, you can always turn the face briefly around.

Whatever you do, *don't* focus directly on time itself during the presleep interval. It is a self-defeating behavior, and will inhibit the very behavior you want to induce: falling asleep.

COLORS

Use Colors in Your Bedroom That Tend to Induce Relaxation. The colors of the visible portion of the electromagnetic spectrum are red, orange, yellow, green, blue, indigo, and violet. (The *electromagnetic spectrum* itself is made up of electromagnetic waves including X-rays, infrared, and ultraviolet. These are invisible to the naked eye.) The waves that induce the sensation of red are 700 nanometers in length. (A nanometer is one billionth of a meter.) The waves that induce the sensation of violet are 400 nanometers in length. Red waves are said to be "long." And violet waves are said to be "short."

Research on the psychological effect of color suggests that waves from the long end of the visible spectrum—red, orange, and yellow—tend to excite the nervous system. They increase arousal by clicking on the sympathetic division of your autonomic nervous system. On the other hand, waves from the short end of the visible spectrum—green, blue, indigo, and violet—tend to calm the nervous system. They decrease arousal by clicking on the parasympathetic division of your autonomic nervous system.

You want your bedroom to have a tranquilizing effect. Consequently, it makes sense decorate the bedroom in colors that induce relaxation. Although you may only spend a short time in the bedroom with the lights on before you go to sleep, you don't want to be hit with a blast of stimulating color just before you settle down.

Whenever you go in and out of your bedroom, you don't want its colors to increase alertness. If they do, then increased alertness will become a conditioned response associated with the bedroom. When you step into your bedroom just before retiring, you will automatically tend to awaken instead of getting drowsy. This is clearly undesirable and antagonistic to the sleep you seek.

DEHYDRATION

Be Sure That Your Body Is Not Somewhat Dehydrated. It is logical to assume that your inborn thirst drive is a reliable guide to how much water you should consume. However, quite a few people don't drink enough water. The reasons for this are several, ranging from medical problems to the way in which a given person's hypothalamus functions. People who don't take in sufficient amounts of water may suffer from mild dehydration. This condition can be a factor in several problems including constipation and migraine headaches. It can also be a factor in insomnia. In order to counteract nighttime dehydration it is a good idea to drink a full eight-ounce glass of water, or the equivalent in milk, decaffeinated coffee, or caffeine-free herbal tea within a one-hour period before retiring. (Some people argue that a glass or cup of these beverages is not equivalent to a glass of clear water. This is incorrect. The bulk of all three of them is simply water.)

Resistance to drinking the equivalent of a full glass of water shortly before retiring is often expressed in the protest, "But then I'll have to get up and go to the bathroom during the night." That's right. And, oddly, even if you are somewhat dehydrated your kidneys will produce urine, and you'll have to get up anyway. You might not void quite as much if you're somewhat dehydrated, but this is obviously of no advantage.

DOUBLE-CHECKING

If You Feel a Strong Desire to Double-Check Locks and Electrical Appliances, By All Means Do So. Sabrina L. says, "My husband laughs at me. After I'm in bed, I often think, 'I wonder if the back door is locked. Or, I wonder if I unplugged the iron.' One part of me says, 'Of course the back door is locked.' Another part of me says, 'I'm not so sure.' So I usually get up and go double-check. Usually everything's OK because I *did* make a first check ten minutes before. However, you know what? Two or three times a year I *do* find an unlocked door, an iron plugged in, or the coffee maker switch in the "On" position. So I feel vindicated."

Don't be too quick to label yourself "obsessive-compulsive." Feeling secure at night is an important factor in obtaining better sleep. So *do* get up and go double-check if you really want to. Redundant action is one way we can feel sure that something has really been done.

ENTERTAINING YOURSELF

Acquire the Art of Entertaining Yourself in Bed. One of the factors associated with behavioral insomnia is simple boredom. In the presleep interval many people are bored. Two minutes seems like five minutes or more. Actually, it is completely normal to spend as much as from ten to twenty minutes in bed before falling asleep. If you are a strong-willed personality with a lot of projects, someone who is quite active during the day, you may subjectively experience the presleep interval as somewhat longer than it objectively is.

The art of entertaining yourself can be acquired. This will greatly reduce boredom during the presleep interval and allow you to remain in bed without feeling too restless. Angelo G. says, "I know forty or fifty popular songs by heart—words and music. I've found that I can 'play'

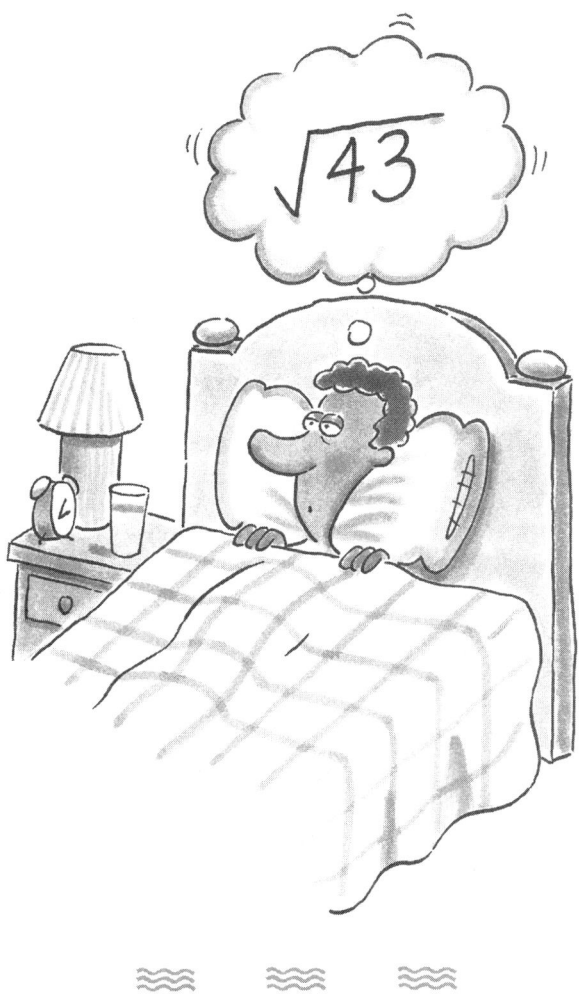

the songs in my head pretty much at will. It's somewhat like putting on tapes. I 'listen' to some of my favorite songs, and, without realizing it, at some point I fall asleep."

Rhonda P. says, "I don't know how many movies I've seen—hundreds I guess. When I get bored in bed I simply pick a favorite movie and 'run' it on a mental screen.

I call this 'my theater of the mind.' I'm not bored. The time passes easily, and soon I'm fast asleep."

Ambrose G. says, "I give myself moderately challenging mental tasks. For example, I will try to name as many of the fifty states as I can. Or I will try to think of as many presidents of the United States as I can. Or I will try to multiply a one-digit number by a two-digit number such as seven times twenty-two. I don't want to get hung up. So if a task seems too complicated, I say, 'to heck with it.' This approach seems to work for me."

If you are a person who is easily bored, you will find it useful to explore ways of mentally entertaining yourself, ways that are compatible with your own personality and interests, while you are waiting to fall asleep.

FANS

Use the Hum of a Fan to Mask Distracting Sounds. Many people find that the hum of a fan helps them to fall asleep. The constant sound not only masks distracting sounds, it also provides a steady source of auditory stimulation that is likely to induce a state of sleep. A running electric motor is a source of white noise. The noise is called "white" because in contains a random mixture of sound waves. (The concept of white noise is adapted from the physics of light; white light contains a random mixture of the electromagnetic waves that produce color sensations.)

A common objection to the use of the sound of a fan to induce sleep, is that the breeze coming from the fan is an irritant. If so, turn the fan away from you, toward a wall. This will help circulate the air in the room and the fan won't blow directly on you. The same advice applies to overhead ceiling fans. They can be switched to a reverse position, and the air will blow upwards toward the ceiling. Also, if you are looking primarily for the hum, set the switch on the "Low" position.

HOME SECURITY SYSTEMS

If You Feel Threatened by the Possibility of Intruders, Obtain a Home Security System. A high-quality home security system will make you feel safer in your own home, particularly at night. You will feel protected and less vulnerable. Although most systems have some drawbacks, shop around and find one that suits your needs. If you are in constant fear that a stranger may invade your territory, it is nearly impossible to relax and go to sleep.

And be sure that you take advantage of commonsense precautions. Have dead bolts on your doors and a way of locking windows. These simple safeguards will help you sleep more soundly.

HYPNAGOGIC REVERIE

Learn to Enjoy Hypnagogic Reverie. Hypnagogic reverie is associated with a normal stage of borderline consciousness between full consciousness and sleep. It occurs commonly during the presleep interval. The word *hypnagogic* is related to the word *hypnosis*.

When you are in a state of hypnagogic reverie your mind spontaneously produces vivid "sights" and "sounds." Sometimes there are near-hallucinations—sights, sounds, and other perceptions—that seem almost real. If you have these experiences from time to time, don't be upset. They are not considered to be pathological by psychiatry and clinical psychology. On the contrary, the experiences linked to hypnagogic reverie are normal expressions arising from a subconscious level. Like dreams, they are manifestations, sometimes in symbolical form, of emotional conflicts and wishes.

Just relax and enjoy the highly lucid experiences you have during hypnagogic reverie. Carleton E. says, "For many months, off and on, I used to have this fantastic image of myself sitting on a winged horse just as I was getting drowsy and about to fall asleep. Something about the whole thing upset me and I would find myself fighting the image and waking up. Then one night I decided to go with it. Half-conscious, I took control of the image and creatively spun it out to its logical conclusion. I found myself riding the winged horse to the moon. When I landed, I got off of the horse. A beautiful woman in a sheer white gown approached me. Without a word, we embraced and kissed. And then the image evaporated like a soap bubble. I decided that the woman on the moon represents my ideal, the woman I hope to meet someday. Whatever it means, I've learned to enjoy this, and other, fantasies when they occur. They don't disturb me now. Instead, they tend to relax me and help me to fall asleep."

MATTRESSES

Be Sure That You Are Sleeping on a Mattress That Is Right for You. A great deal of misinformation surrounds the whole subject of mattresses. People who suffer from insomnia are easy prey for salespersons who make all sorts of extravagant claims about the way in which a particular mattress "keeps the spine straight," or "allows for a minimum of pressure on the joints," and so forth. And the price you pay for a mattress is not a reliable criterion. Sometimes people pay as much as two times more than they need to for a mattress that will serve them no better than a less expensive one.

Usually you are told that the mattress should be "firm," that this gives you better support. It is certainly true that if you use an old broken down mattress with feeble springs, it will be hard on your back. But should you buy a mattress that is marked "firm" if you only weigh 110 pounds? Under such circumstances, you might feel as if you are sleeping on a slab of granite. If you don't weigh much, a mattress that is marked "medium" might be better. On the other hand, if you are obese, a mattress that is marked "extrafirm" will probably be better for you.

Note that I have used the word *marked* above, not *rated*. A manufacturer's markings are not certified ratings. Be sure you follow the old principle of caveat emptor, or "buyer beware." You have to recline on a mattress in a number of positions, including on your side, in order to make your own personal rating of "soft," "medium," "firm," or "extrafirm." You can only do this if you have shopped around and tried out more than one mattress.

Sometimes when a couple sleeps on the same mattress there can be a problem if they are of different weights. One or both persons may feel uncomfortable. For example, a husband might feel a mattress is too soft and his wife might be convinced that the same mattress is too hard. In a case like this it is probably a good idea to obtain separate mattresses for each individual.

What about putting a board under your bed? This advice is often given to people who have back complaints. I contend that a board is generally too rigid and unyielding. Using a board is based on the idea that one's mattress is too soft or broken down. It is probably a better idea to sleep on an extrafirm mattress than to put a board under an old, or a soft, mattress.

NAPS

If at All Possible, Take an Afternoon Nap. Think about the comic strip character Dagwood Bumstead. He is frequently shown taking a nap on the living room sofa. Is he just lazy, or is he observing a deep biological program? The evidence is in favor of the latter interpretation. Sleep research has shown that the circadian rhythm of most people has a natural letdown phase between approximately 1:00 P.M. to 4:00 P.M. If you can take a nap lasting from as little as ten to twenty minutes within this time frame, it can be wonderfully refreshing and do much to combat sleep deprivation. Although there are exceptions, in most cases it is a good idea to limit afternoon naps to about half an hour. More napping may interfere with nighttime sleep.

True, your schedule and work conditions might not allow you to take a nap. But sometimes we can adapt to situations more readily than we at first believe we can. Linette W., a community college instructor, says, "I sometimes doze off in my office chair for about ten or fifteen minutes in the afternoon. I generally lock the door." Dan H., an insurance underwriter, says, "I have about a forty-minute drive home every day. I get off work at 4:00 P.M. and often take a nap in the car before I drive home. After I wake up, I stop and get a cup of coffee." Explore your own options.

Some people say that a nap leaves them feeling dull and sluggish. And this does seem to be true for some individuals. If you get enough sleep during the night, a nap may not be very important. On the other hand, the sluggish feeling immediately following a nap is often brief. That is why Dan H., referred to above, has a cup of coffee before he drives home. The long run effect of naps on your mental and emotional well being is usually positive.

NEGATIVE PRACTICE

Use Negative Practice to Combat a Restless Legs Syndrome. A common symptom associated with insomnia is the *restless legs syndrome*. The victim's legs make involuntary jerky motions while the individual tries to go to sleep. The more the victim tries to inhibit the involuntary motions, the worse they get. If you suffer from this syndrome, you should first be assured by a physician that you do not suffer from a neurological problem. Assuming that this is not your problem, a restless legs syndrome responds well to a behavioral strategy known as *negative practice*.

Negative practice was formulated a number of years ago by the psychologist Knight Dunlap. And it is of particular value in the extinction (breaking) of maladaptive motor habits. Such habits include nail biting, tics, certain features of stuttering, and the restless legs syndrome.

Negative practice requires that the individual *voluntarily* practice the error. For example, a person with a nail biting problem can stand in front of a mirror for five minute sessions twice a day and go through all of the motor movements involved in nail biting. (In this case the individual does not actually have to bite the nails.) This brings the previously involuntary behavior under voluntary control. This is a new experience for a person with a maladaptive motor habit. Usually one is unsuccessfully trying to inhibit, not make manifest, the habit.

So, silly as it sounds, if you suffer from a restless legs syndrome, spend about three or four minutes in a comfortable chair *voluntarily* jerking your legs. Mimic the motions you actually make when you cannot rest. This voluntary action will automatically inhibit the tendency toward involuntary action later when you are in bed. If the restless legs syndrome appears, get out of bed, go to the comfortable chair, and engage in voluntary leg movements again. Then return to bed.

Don't do the voluntary motions in bed. You want to get conditioned to think of your bed as a place where this does *not* happen.

NIGHT-LIGHTS

Keep a Night-Light on in a Bathroom or the Hallway. It makes both children and adults feel more secure to have just a little light available when they wake up in the middle of the night. And more than emotional security is involved. A night-light keeps us from stubbing our toes or otherwise bumping into things. It is doubtful that a small indirect light will inhibit the secretion of melatonin to any significant degree.

NIGHTCAPS

Wear a Nightcap to Bed. The word *nightcap* has two meanings. Nowadays the first meaning that probably comes to mind is a drink containing alcohol that is sipped just before going to bed. As indicated in chapter 2, this kind of a sleeping potion is of doubtful long-term value. However, a second and original meaning of a nightcap is a head covering worn in bed. Almost 175 years ago Clement Moore referred to wearing a cap to bed in his well-known poem "A Visit from St. Nicholas." (This poem is also known as "'Twas the Night Before Christmas.") The "cap" being referred to is a nightcap. He also indicates that "Ma" was wearing a "kerchief." This meant that his wife was also wearing a head covering. Charles Dickens's *A Christmas Carol* was published twenty years after Moore's poem. Illustrations of Scrooge in bed usually show him wearing a big nightcap.

The practice of wearing a nightcap to bed seems to have faded away. This is probably because with the advent of thermostats and forced-air ducts homes are more well heated at night then they used to be. Nonetheless, a common cause of sleep restlessness is a cold head. If one's hair is thin, or if circulation to the scalp is slightly inadequate, the top of one's head may be chilled. A simple correction is to wear a nightcap or a kerchief. (Contemporary apparel can consist of a soft, knitted cap.)

It is not only the head that can be cold. Any of the extremities, meaning the head, hands, and feet, are prone to coldness because they are farther from the heart than the rest of the body. (They are called "extremities" because they are an "extreme" distance from the heart.) It takes circulating blood to create natural warmth in a limb. If your feet tend to be cold, wear socks to bed. If your hands tend to be cold, keep them under the covers. If this solution is inadequate, consider wearing gloves or mittens to bed.

PILLOWS

Be Sure That You Are Happy with Your Pillow. It may seem obvious that you should be happy with your pillow. But, amazingly, there are people who put up with pillows

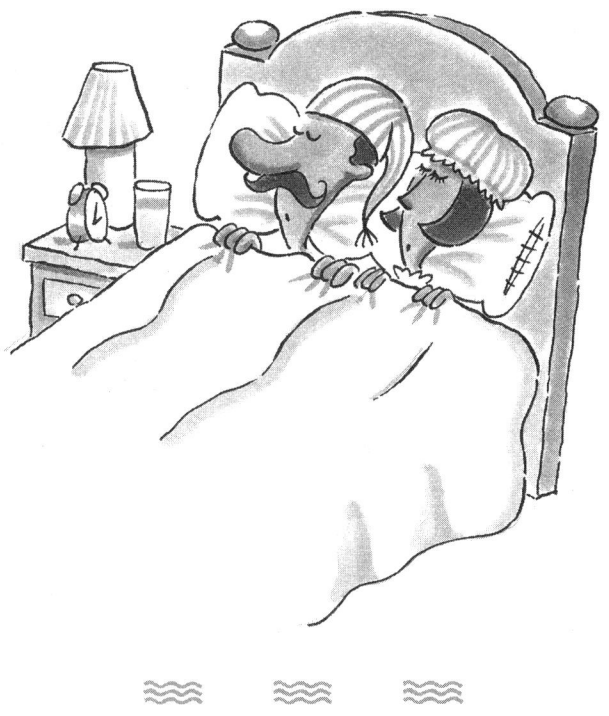

that they don't like for months and even years. If you don't like your pillow, *get rid of it!*

Pillows, like mattresses, can be too hard and too soft. But it's all a matter of personal preference. Sometimes when a pillow is stuffed with an animal substance such as down or feathers you may have a bit of an allergic reaction. Unexplained sneezing or wheezing often aggravates insomnia. (See the section headed "Allergens.") If you suspect that this might be a problem, obtain a pillow made of a synthetic material. If your pillow seems to give you a pain in the neck (literally!), you can obtain a special therapeutic pillow designed to give you better head support. Talk this over with a physician or a pharmacist. Stores that specialize in home medical equipment can also be good sources of information.

Experienced travelers recommend that when you travel, if at all possible, take your pillow with you. It can make all the difference between restlessness and a good night's sleep.

SEPARATE BEDROOMS

Under Certain Conditions, It Is a Good Idea to Have Separate Bedrooms. In the early years of a marriage a couple will almost certainly not want to have even separate beds, let alone separate bedrooms. Nonetheless, as time passes, sometimes a person finds that the sleep idiosyncrasies of a partner interfere with his or her own sleep. Regina L. has been married for twenty-four years to the same man. She says, "I married Burton when he was twenty-four and I was twenty-two. We were starry eyed and madly in love. He was in the navy and we had a little apartment. We slept like two peas in a pod in a double bed, snuggled up, and loved every minute of it. Ten years later we were sleeping in a king-size bed and irritated each other once in a while. Now Burton is fifty pounds overweight, snores, turns heavily, and pulls the bedclothes off of me. He complains that I talk in my sleep and smack my lips at night. He wants the bedroom about ten degrees cooler than I want it. Let's face it. We still love each other, and we have our moments, but we're incompatible sleeping partners. About two years ago we decided to sleep in separate bedrooms. We're both happier, getting along better, and obtaining some decent sleep. Interestingly, it has made our relationship more erotic, rather than less. When we get together in the same bed now it's sort of special."

Face facts. If you have the space in your home, and if separate bedrooms will help you and your partner get a good night's sleep, then don't let pride stand in your way. Don't think, "I guess we don't love each other any more." Maybe agreeing to sleep in separate bedrooms is one of the most considerate and loving things you can do for each other.

SLEEP PATTERNS

Learn to Accept an Idiosyncratic Sleep Pattern. Chapter 2 described a normal sleep pattern. This is the pattern typical of the average person. An *idiosyncratic sleep pattern* is the pattern that is characteristic of you as a unique individual. It can deviate significantly from the normal pattern and still be a healthful one.

Person 1 says, "I go to bed at midnight. I fall asleep within ten minutes and I sleep like a log until 5:00 A.M. Then I get up, feel good all day, and don't have a need for a nap. My wife says I'm sleep deprived. If I am, I'm not aware of it."

Person 2 says, "I get sleepy around 8:00 P.M. If we're not out for the evening or entertaining, I sleep in my recliner until about 10:00 P.M. Then I'm awake again until about 12:30 A.M. I force myself to go the bed and usually have a little trouble falling asleep. But when I do, I tend to sleep soundly until I get up in the morning."

Person 3 says, "I get up and go to the bathroom two or three times during the night. But I always go back to sleep easily."

Person 4 says, "Almost every night around 2:00 A.M. I have to get up and read for about half an hour. Then it's OK. I can go back to bed and sleep again."

Person 5 says, "I sleep four or five hours every night. But I'm really sleepy in the afternoon. Fortunately, my life style allows me to take a big two hour-nap every afternoon. I've been doing this for years."

All of these people have idiosyncratic sleep patterns. They don't fit an idealized image of how and when to sleep. Nonetheless, there is no pathology. Even in the case of Person 1 there may be no problem. A few people, very few, can thrive on as little as five hours of sleep in a twenty-four-hour period. There are, on the other hand, some people who need as much as a total of ten hours in order to function effectively.

You have to know yourself, your own needs and your own individual traits. If your sleep pattern isn't quite like that of most other people, there is nothing to worry about if it is compatible with your own personality and life style. Don't define yourself as suffering from insomnia just because your behavior differs from that of others.

TRANSITIONAL OBJECTS

Consider Providing Yourself with a Transitional Object. A *transitional object* is usually defined as an object to which a child is attached such as a blanket, a particular pillow, or a teddy bear. We all know that such objects make children feel secure and help them to go to sleep. The word *transitional* is used to describe the object because attachment to it is not, of course, supposed to be permanent. It provides a bridge from the world of the child to the world of the adult.

But adults, like children, have their insecurities. The child self in you still experiences fear and anxiety. If this were not so, tranquilizers, also known as *antianxiety agents*, would not be so popular.

As foolish at it may at first seem, a transitional object can often help an adult sleep. It need not be as obvious as a blanket. Garrett A. says, "One day I remembered that when I was a child I always wanted to go to sleep with my Mickey Mouse watch on. I thought to myself, Why not? And I went to a store and bought one. I like to wear it to bed. Just putting it on helps me relax and go to sleep."

Gloriane L. says, "When I was a child I really enjoyed A. A. Milne's books *Winnie-the-Pooh* and *The House at Pooh Corner*. Recently I bought both books for my permanent collection."

Ilene M. says, "When I was a child I always went to sleep hugging a little pink pillow. I bought a pillow similar to the original one the other day, and I use it as a 'snuggle thing' sometimes."

Percy F. says, "Bugs Bunny is my hero. What a guy! I keep an old Bugs Bunny comic book in the bottom

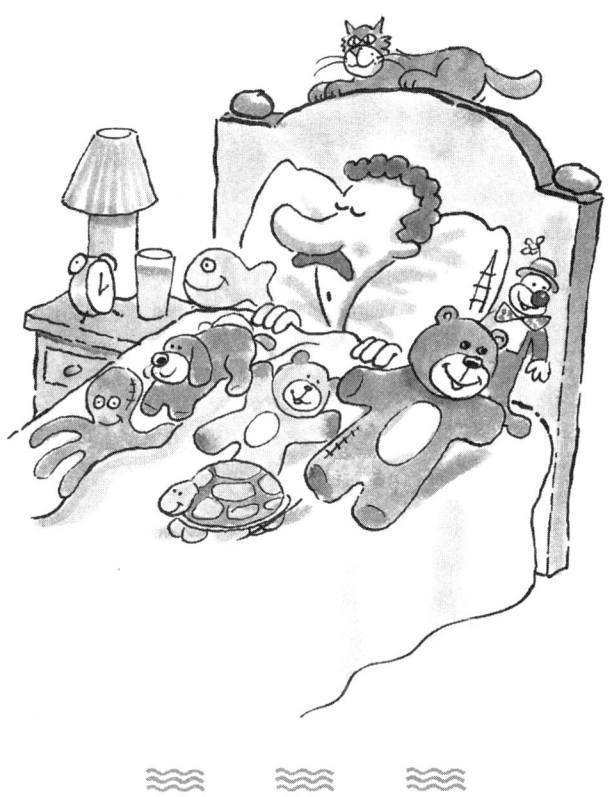

drawer of my bed stand. I seldom look at it, but I kind of like knowing that it's there."

If a transitional object will provide comfort to your child self and help you sleep, then you might consider allowing yourself this small personal indulgence.

UNCONVENTIONAL SLEEPING PLACES

Give Yourself Permission to Sleep in an Unconventional Place. There is no rule that says you have to do all of your sleeping in bed in your bedroom. Dana P. says, "I wake up most mornings about 4:00 A.M. and find it difficult to go back to sleep in bed. But the recliner in the family room sounds good. I put on my robe, cover my lap and legs with a blanket, and sleep like a baby for two more hours."

Rita D. says, "I fall asleep around 10:00 P.M. in front of the television most nights, and often don't wake until around 1:00 A.M. I've had three hours of good sleep, and I make an easy transition to my bed. For years I thought there was something 'wrong' with this pattern. But what's wrong with it if I like it and it works for me?"

If you enjoy spending part of the night sleeping on a sofa, a recliner, or on a second bed, give yourself permission to be an individual. There is no stereotyped pattern that you have to follow. What *is* important is that you be happy and that you get some high-quality sleep.

WATER BEDS

If You Find It Difficult to Rest on a Conventional Mattress, Consider Using a Water Bed. A water bed is actually a special kind of mattress. It is a thick rectangular bag, and is often made of vinyl. When the bag is filled with an optimal amount of water, it provides a sleeping surface. Some people find water beds remarkably comfortable. Others complain that they feel insecure on them; they don't feel properly supported. This is a sensation that may go away with repeated use.

The main virtue of water beds is that they are devoid of pressure points. Support for the body is evenly distributed. Consequently, water beds are useful to treat persons suffering from burns. They also help bed-bound persons to avoid getting bed sores.

If you are afflicted with quite a few aches and pains in your muscles and joints, a water bed may provide you with significant relief. Ameila H. says, "I suffer from rheumatoid arthritis, and I can only spend a few hours at a time in a conventional bed. The discomfort becomes unbearable. But I rest comfortably on a water bed. It takes all of the pressure off of my joints, and it has been a real blessing."

The Last Word

You don't, of course, have to use all, or even the majority, of suggestions in this chapter in order to have a beneficial impact on your own sleep process. You need only pick and choose the tips and techniques that appeal to you, that you suspect might work in your particular case. And experiment. Vary the suggestions so that they fit your own personality. The recommendations offered in this chapter are like ready-made clothes on the rack. In order to wear them comfortably, they may need a little alteration.

Assuming that you suffer from behavioral insomnia, it is fairly certain that the information provided in the prior pages, if applied with patience and an open attitude, can help you to rid yourself of some of your worst symptoms.

Key Points to Remember

- There are many ways to cope with behavioral insomnia. What works for one person will not work for another.
- This chapter provided a "catalog" of sleep-inducing tips and techniques that work for many people.
- For convenient reference, the suggestions have been arranged in alphabetical order.
- Vary the suggestions so that they fit your own personality.

8 PROFESSIONAL ASSISTANCE: MEDICAL TREATMENTS AND PSYCHOTHERAPY

There is much that you can do for yourself if your problem is behavioral insomnia. This book has given you a number of self-directed coping strategies that are likely to be highly effective.

Nonetheless, there are times when one may feel overwhelmed by the symptoms of a sleep disorder. An individual may recognize that the problem exceeds his or her general knowledge and coping abilities. If such is the case for you, then it is time to turn to professional assistance.

Medical Treatments

There is much that physicians can do to effectively help persons suffering from sleep disorders. (Keep in mind that psychiatrists are physicians. Psychiatry is a medical specialty.)

You will recall from chapter I that *symptomatic insomnia* is insomnia that is secondary to a medical problem. In the case of this kind of insomnia it is essential to treat the underlying organic disturbance. *Sleep apnea* and *narcolepsy*, also discussed in chapter I, provide two more examples of sleep disorders that are associated with disturbed biological processes.

SURGERY

Surgery for a sleep disorder? At first the concept seems absurd. How is cutting into the body going to make a person sleep better?

The first and most obvious instance where surgery is sometimes helpful is in the treatment of *sleep apnea* (a temporary cessation of breathing). There is a category of sleep apnea known as *obstructive sleep apnea*. This is sometimes caused primarily by the movement of the uvula and other flaccid tissue toward the rear of the throat. (The *uvula* is a part of the soft palate and hangs like a pendant.) In some instances a *tracheostomy* is recommended. This is a procedure that enlarges the windpipe, making breathing easier. Surgery is, not, of course, the only treatment for sleep apnea. Practical strategies that may help the individual avoid surgery include losing weight, reducing overall stress, stopping smoking, and restricting alcohol.

An additional practical strategy that may be of value in a self-help approach to sleep apnea is to sew a tennis ball into the back of one's pajamas. This will automatically restrain the individual from sleeping on his or her back. In some cases, sleep apnea will diminish greatly if the person can learn to consistently sleep on one side or the other.

Here are some examples of medical conditions that can cause or aggravate insomnia: bunions, carpal-tunnel syndrome, blockages in the coronary arteries, a protruding intervertebral disk (a "ruptured" disk), duodenal ulcer, enlarged prostate gland, gallstones, hemorrhoids, hiatal hernia, infected tear duct, infected tooth, ingrown toenail, nasal polyps, peptic ulcer, periodontal ("gum") infection, and varicose veins. All of these problems may respond to either significant surgery or modest surgical interventions, depending on the nature and the severity of the condition.

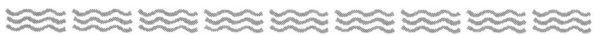

DRUG THERAPY

Drug therapy for sleep disorders tends to take advantage of three classes of drugs: (1) antihistamines; (2) antianxiety agents; and (3) barbiturates.

Antihistamines are drugs that are used to diminish symptoms associated with allergic reactions (for example, sneezing and difficulty in breathing). They work by hindering the activity of *histamine*, a substance released by cells when they have an adverse reaction to allergens. If upper respiratory problems are interfering with your rest, antihistamines can help you breath more freely, and this in turn helps you to sleep. An extra dividend associated with antihistamines is that they tend to make a person drowsy.

Consequently, they are sometimes marketed primarily as over-the-counter sleeping pills. As you can see from the prior statement, antihistamines are available in low doses without a prescription. Larger doses require a prescription.

Antianxiety agents, as their name suggests, reduce anxiety. They accomplish this by relaxing the muscles; this in turn induces lowered central nervous system arousal. And such lowered arousal is physiologically incompatible with anxiety. These drugs are also classified as "minor tranquilizers" and "sedative-hypnotic agents." Their sedative-hypnotic effect also makes them a useful ingredient in sleeping pills. Although they are not considered to be highly addictive from a physiological standpoint, they are potentially psychologically addictive. This simply means that people tend to get dependent on them. These agents require a prescription.

Barbiturates are powerful sedatives for which a prescription is required. They lower central nervous system arousal, having an effect that is somewhat similar to alcohol. They induce sleep, but are not prescribed as often as they used to be. The antianxiety agents are now more likely to be prescribed. Barbiturates are addictive at a physiological level and have a significant potential for abuse.

Drug therapy is not a cure for insomnia. It is a treatment, and its value resides mainly in helping a person cope with occasional, not chronic, insomnia. Drugs have varying degrees of adverse side effects. Also, there is a phenomenon known as *drug tolerance*. After a drug has been taken on a regular basis for a given period of time it produces less and less of the effect that it was intended to produce. Drugs have their place in the treatment of sleep disorders. But they should be used sparingly and judiciously.

You will recall from chapter 2 the point was made that sleeping pills can sometimes interfere with rapid eye movement (REM) sleep. Consequently, sometimes they are counterproductive.

TREATMENTS FOR RESPIRATORY PROBLEMS

Respiratory problems such as abnormal breathing, coughing, wheezing, sneezing, and the inability to take deep breaths can be significant factors in insomnia. Principal treatments for these kinds of problems include: (1) allergen desensitization therapy; (2) drug therapy; and (3) respiratory therapy.

Allergen desensitization therapy consists of first testing the individual for allergens that interfere with normal breathing. Then one is given small subcutaneous amounts of the allergen over a period of time. This will often lead to *desensitization*, an inability of the allergen to induce its adverse reaction. Allergen desensitization therapy is conducted by an *allergist*, a physician who specializes in the treatment of allergies.

Drug therapy for respiratory problems includes the use of various medications designed to provide upper respiratory relief. Two key kinds of drugs used are antihistamines and epinephrine. *Antihistamines*, discussed earlier, reduce some of the more severe symptoms of allergies.

Epinephrine is a drug that stimulates the heart. It also opens up airways. The drug can be delivered in either pill form or with the use of an inhaler. The drugs identified can be purchased over the counter in low dosages. In larger dosages, a prescription is required.

Inhalation therapy is characterized by such procedures as the administration of medication through a *nebulizer*, a device that acts as a pump. Wearing a face mask, the patient is able to obtain substantial amounts of drugs that ease breathing. *Breathing exercises* provide another mode of inhalation therapy. Inhalation therapy is conducted by paramedical personnel with special training. This kind of therapy requires a physician's prescription.

ENDOCRINE THERAPY

Endocrine therapy involves the administration of hormones to alleviate certain medical conditions. Three examples of such conditions that can interfere with normal sleep are diabetes, hypothyroidism, and premenstrual stress syndrome (PMS). *Diabetes* is characterized by abnormal levels of glucose in the blood. When blood sugar is too high it may be difficult to sleep. When it is too low it may be difficult to stay awake. Diabetes is often treated with *insulin*, a hormone that regulates blood sugar.

Hypothyroidism occurs when the thyroid gland does not produce enough of its hormone, thyroxin. If a person has what is informally termed a "sluggish thyroid gland," the individual will lack "get up and go." Also, he or she may suffer from *hypersomnia*, difficulty in staying awake (see chapter 1). Hypothyroidism can be treated with *thyroxine*, a prescription drug that boosts the metabolic rate.

Premenstrual stress syndrome (PMS) is characterized by a group of symptoms including cramps, headaches, anxiety, depression, and insomnia. Antianxiety drugs, antidepressant drugs, and estrogen hormones are often prescribed for PMS.

LIFESTYLE THERAPY

A strong emerging trend among physicians is called *behavioral medicine*. It is now generally recognized that the patient's own behavior is a principal factor in the treatment of chronic illnesses. For example, a person with diabetes may respond to insulin. But he or she also is advised to make dietary modifications. Or, a person who has had heart bypass surgery may be told that he or she should restrict saturated fats in the diet, stop smoking, and take some regular, moderate aerobic exercise.

Your own lifestyle has a lot to do with the way in which you sleep. Physicians and psychologists will often make highly specific recommendations concerning your diet, exercise, and sleep habits. These interventions obviously do not involve either surgery or drugs, but they can be highly effective in the treatment of the sleep disorders. They tend to be highly similar to the kinds of suggestions made in the prior chapters of the book.

Lifestyle therapy is a kind of therapy that requires *your* involvement and commitment. It is not really something that can be done *to* you. You have to do it for yourself. However, the knowledge and experience of professional persons can be very helpful in guiding you and indicating *what* you should do.

Psychotherapy

Psychotherapy approaches the treatment of sleep disorders from the point of view of behavioral factors such as motivational dispositions, emotional states, thoughts, perceptions, and habits. Its greatest value is in the treatment of *behavioral insomnia*, a kind of insomnia that has no organic pathology associated with it. This kind of insomnia has been a principal focus of this book. If behavioral insomnia is chronic, and if efforts to use this book's suggestions on your own have met with limited success, then it is time to explore psychotherapy.

Let's define *psychotherapy* as a healing of the self through the use of psychological principles. An informal name for psychotherapy is "the talking cure."

If you decide to seek psychotherapy, it is essential that you assure yourself that your therapist is a fully qualified person. He or she should hold a state license and be certified by a board of examiners. Three kinds of professional persons are qualified to practice psychotherapy: (1) psychiatrists; (2) clinical psychologists; and (3) clinical social workers.

Below you will find various approaches to psychotherapy. These approaches are not mutually exclusive. They can be combined to create an effective treatment program. The skilled therapist is familiar with all of the approaches. Contemporary psychotherapy is said to be *multimodal*, meaning more than one mode of therapy is often used with a given client. (The term *eclectic* is also sometimes used to describe the general viewpoint of a therapist who is open to several approaches.)

THE PSYCHODYNAMIC APPROACH

The *psychodynamic approach* assumes that human beings have an unconscious mental life. This approach has its roots in classical psychoanalysis, the kind of psychotherapy pioneered by Sigmund Freud. Although today classical psychoanalysis is certainly not the only, or even the principal, mode of therapy, it occupies a unique place in the history of psychotherapy. It is the first of the modern approaches to psychotherapy.

Unconscious mental life arises from a tendency in the mind to repress certain memories, ideas, and wishes. It is as if an invisible hand in the mind shoves down selected information to a psychological nether land. What kind of mental content is likely to get repressed? The most likely candidates are emotionally traumatic childhood memories and forbidden wishes. The banished wishes tend to be of an aggressive or sexual nature. They are offensive in terms of one's particular moral code.

The psychodynamic approach assumes that the self is a battlefield of conflicting emotions. If repression is incomplete, if there is a substantial amount of unfinished emotional business in your life, it is likely to interfere with your ability to sleep. In Freud's approach to dream interpretation, it is the effort of the repressed material to express itself that produces fantastic dreams. (See chapter 4).

Taking a psychodynamic approach, your therapist will help you explore the unconscious aspects of your mental life. This can be done through dream interpretation. It can also be done through a technique called *free association* in which you are encouraged to talk more or less at random about your life. Seemingly arbitrary mental connections often reveal a great deal about one's emotional conflicts.

The psychodynamic approach is a profound one. It seeks to help you resolve long-standing emotional problems that may be persistent factors contributing to behavioral insomnia.

THE BEHAVIORAL APPROACH

The *behavioral approach* is based on the assumption that behavior, both adaptive and maladaptive, is learned. *Learning* is defined as a more or less permanent change in behavior, or a behavioral tendency, as a result of experience. The behavioral approach in psychology is associated with the findings of researchers such as Ivan Pavlov, John B. Watson, and B. F. Skinner. Although these individuals were not psychotherapists, their understandings and findings have been used extensively in modern therapy.

The behavioral approach is obviously well suited to treat behavioral insomnia. Behavioral insomnia is to a large extent a phenomenon of learning. Maladaptive ways of responding to a natural need, sleep, can be looked upon as principal sources of the sufferer's problem. There is much hope in the behavioral approach because it is assumed that what has been learned can be unlearned. We are all familiar with the idea of "breaking" a habit. The formal name for this in the psychology of learning is "extinction." *Extinction* is the unlearning of a habit. If a habit cannot be extinguished, sometimes it can be modified. The maladaptive habit is not completely gone, but it has been changed in such a way that it no longer presents a significant problem to the individual.

Taking a behavioral approach, your psychotherapist will help you either extinguish or modify the kinds of habits that contribute to behavioral insomnia. The behavioral approach is very practical. It is specific and deals with the *here* and the *now*. It is not so concerned with the *why* of a problem as the *how* of its satisfactory resolution.

THE COGNITIVE APPROACH

The *cognitive approach* in psychotherapy assumes that irrational thoughts often induce emotional distress. Two therapists who have contributed much to this approach are Albert Ellis and Aaron Beck. *Irrational thoughts*, a term employed by Ellis, are maladaptive in nature. They do not accurately reflect reality, but seem to. Such thoughts are based on *cognitive distortions*, tendencies of the mind to make hasty generalizations or overuse either/or logic. These thoughts tend to be involuntary, and we often engage in them with a minimum of reflection and analysis. (Beck uses the term *automatic thoughts* to capture the involuntary aspect of the kinds of thoughts that are likely to create emotional difficulties.)

As indicated in earlier chapters, the anxiety and depression generated by irrational thoughts can interfere with normal sleep.

Taking a cognitive approach, your therapist will encourage you to challenge your own irrational thoughts, to examine the assumptions on which they are based. If you can think more realistically and constructively about your life and the world, you will suffer less and less from unnecessary anxiety and depression. And, in turn, you will obtain better sleep.

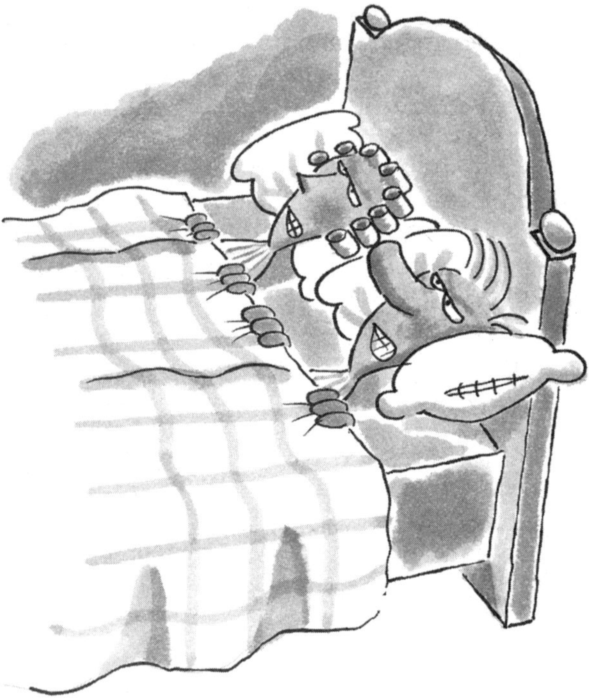

THE INTERPERSONAL APPROACH

The interpersonal approach assumes that many of our personal problems are either caused or aggravated by the way in which we interact with others. In particular, if you have a long-standing relationship with a partner, the way in which the two of you communicate may play an important role in your sleep behavior.

If, for example, the two of you argue just before going to bed, this is likely to induce a bad night's sleep. Or, if your partner wants the room warmer (or cooler) than you want it, you may find it difficult to relax and go to sleep. Other, and similar, examples are given in prior chapters. Taking an interpersonal approach, your therapist will help you and your partner explore more functional ways to interact and establish emotional closeness. The therapist will help you to avoid the kinds of self-defeating games that intimate persons often play. (Ideally, an interactive approach requires the presence in therapy of *both* you and your partner.)

HYPNOTHERAPY

Hypnotherapy refers to the use of hypnosis as a means of alleviating personal problems. *Hypnosis* itself is an altered state of consciousness in which the individual is somewhat more susceptible to suggestions. Chapter 6 was devoted to the subject of self-hypnosis.

Using hypnotherapy, your psychotherapist may help you acquire the art of self-hypnosis. Self-hypnosis, depending on your particular temperament, is a potentially useful tool, a logical procedure that can often help you fall asleep more readily.

Hypnotherapy can also be used to help you break maladaptive habits, the kinds of habits associated with poor sleep hygiene.

BIOFEEDBACK TRAINING

Biofeedback training is a learning procedure in which an electronic apparatus provides high-quality information concerning the momentary state of a natural biological process such as pulse rate, tension in a muscle, brain wave activity, or skin temperature. This kind of training often makes it possible for the individual to gain control of autonomic functions that are traditionally said to be

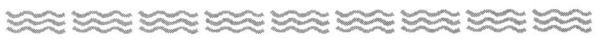

"involuntary." If they *are* involuntary, you are in some cases their victim. On the other hand, when you gain control of these functions, they cross the line from their prior status. They now can be called "voluntary" because *you* are, to some extent, in charge of them.

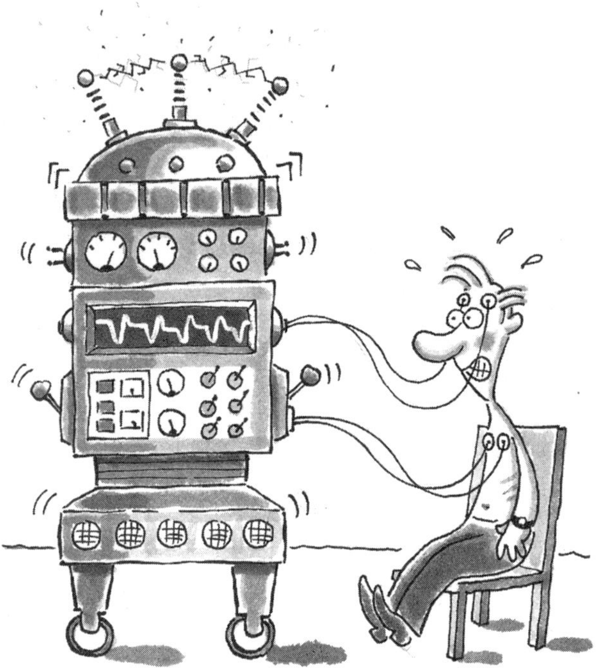

Behavioral insomnia is often associated with an inability to relax. Biofeedback training can be used to induce relaxation in several ways. First, it can be used to help you relax muscles. Muscle relaxation is antagonistic to anxiety, the kind of anxiety that may be keeping you awake.

Second, biofeedback training can be used to induce a higher production of *alpha waves*. Evidence for such waves is provided by electroencephalographic (EEG) recordings; alpha waves occur at the rate of eight to fourteen cycles per second. They are associated with mental relaxation and the presleep stage. The alpha rhythm can be a prelude to the slower *delta waves* associated with deep sleep.

Third, biofeedback training can be used to control headaches. And headaches may interfere with the ability to relax and go to sleep. Tension headaches can be managed by learning to relax the *frontalis*, the forehead muscle.

Migraine headaches, which have a different physiological basis, can be managed by learning to warm the hands. Migraine headaches are often caused by enlarged blood vessels supplying blood to the head and brain. The warming of the hands requires the blood vessels in these extremities to open. This action is antagonistic to the opening of blood vessels in the head area; consequently, warming the hands makes them automatically constrict.

It is, of course, possible to warm the hands without biofeedback training. An often effective home treatment for migraine headaches is to place both hands in a pan of warm water for about ten minutes. You can add to the effectiveness of the treatment by following it with relaxation in a comfortable chair or recliner. The lights should be either off or turned down low. Frequently the addition of a cool compress to the forehead can be helpful. The coolness helps the scalp's blood vessels to constrict.

It is important to note that this procedure is effective with migraine, not tension headaches. It may, in fact, aggravate a tension headache. A tension headache is usually somewhat less severe than a migraine headache. A migraine headache is often accompanied by nausea, weakness, pain on one side of the head, and visual disturbances.

The Last Word

As you can see from the material in this chapter, there is much benefit that can be derived from medical treatment and psychotherapy for the sleep disorders, including chronic behavioral insomnia. There is nothing in professional assistance that contradicts the various tips and techniques given in the prior chapters. On the contrary, professional and self-help approaches are not mutually exclusive, but complementary. In order for an expert's intervention to be effective, the client must *comply* with prescriptions and recommendations. The course of chronic problems such as those associated with the sleep disorders is highly dependent on the individual's lifestyle. And this is under the control of the suffering person, not physicians and clinical psychologists. (Again, keep in mind that psychiatrists, who are highly qualified to treat sleep disorders, are physicians. Psychiatry is a medical specialty.)

Additional information on sleep and the sleep disorders can be obtained by writing to: The National Sleep Foundation, 1367 Connecticut Ave., NW, Dept. SCM, Washington, D.C. 20036.

Key Points to Remember

- There are times when it is important to seek either medical assistance or psychotherapy for a sleep disorder, including behavioral insomnia.
- *Symptomatic insomnia* is insomnia that is secondary to a medical problem.
- Surgery can sometimes be used to treat a sleep disorder.
- Drug therapy for sleep disorders tends to take advantage of three classes of drugs: (1) antihistamines; (2) antianxiety agents; and (3) barbiturates.

- Respiratory problems can be significant factors in insomnia. Principal treatments for these kinds of problems include: (1) allergen desensitization therapy; (2) drug therapy; and (3) respiratory therapy.

- *Endocrine therapy* involves the administration of hormones to alleviate certain medical conditions. Three examples of such conditions that can interfere with normal sleep patterns are diabetes, hypothyroidism, and premenstrual stress syndrome (PMS).

- Your own lifestyle has a lot to do with the way in which you sleep.

- Psychotherapy approaches the treatment of sleep disturbances from the point of view of behavioral factors such as motivational dispositions, emotional states, thoughts, perceptions, and habits.

- The *psychodynamic approach* assumes that human beings have an unconscious mental life.

- The *behavioral approach* is based on the assumption that behavior, both adaptive and maladaptive, is learned.

- The *cognitive approach* assumes that irrational thoughts induce emotional distress.

- The *interpersonal approach* assumes that many of our personal problems are either caused or aggravated by the way in which we interact with others.

- *Hypnotherapy* refers to the use of hypnosis as a means of alleviating personal problems.

- *Biofeedback training* is a learning procedure in which an electronic apparatus provides high-quality information concerning the momentary state of a natural biological process such as pulse rate, tension in a muscle, brain wave activity, or skin temperature.
- There is much benefit that can be derived from medical treatment and psychotherapy for the sleep disorders, including chronic behavioral insomnia.

9 A SEVEN-STEP ANTI-INSOMNIA PROGRAM

You have read *Get a Good Night's Sleep*. You want to make its ideas work for you, but where do you start? First, don't be overwhelmed by a large amount of information. It is all right to be selective, picking out only those ideas that make sense to you in terms of your own unique personality.

Second, feel free to adapt the book's suggestions as you see fit. If a coping strategy has to be modified in some way in order to make it work for you, then tailor it to your needs.

Third, you don't have to do everything at once. You only have to employ a few of the book's tips or techniques at a time in order to get good results.

If the book is really going to help you relax and get a good night's sleep, then just relax about the book itself. Take it and its ideas "slow and easy."

The Weakest Link Approach

A good way to get started in making personal applications from the book is to take the weakest link approach. Think of your maladaptive habits, the kind that keep you from sleeping, as links in a chain. Its a good idea to look for the weakest links and break or modify them first. This will give you a feeling of success and reinforce the belief in your ability to actually improve your sleeping behavior.

Obtain a few index cards. Scan through the chapters, looking for tips and techniques. These are all identified in a distinctive typeface. Jot down six or seven ideas, one to a card, that you believe you can apply readily. Keep the cards in a handy place, and put the self-directed coping strategies to work. As your own ideas and modifications occur to you, add them to the appropriate card.

You should get prompt and effective results from this general approach.

The Seven-Step Program

Assuming that you want to cope with your sleeping difficulties in a systematic way, this section provides a program for doing so.

The book is logical. Each chapter follows the preceding one in a natural sequence. Consequently, it is designed to allow you to make your personal applications in a step-by-step manner.

STEP 1

Turn to chapter 2, "Understanding a Normal Sleep Pattern." This chapter defines states of sleep and explains the characteristics of rapid eye movement (REM) sleep.

Survey the suggestions under the heading "Making Applications." Pick one that seems to be of particular value, and put it to work. Continue in this manner for about one week. Then take Step 2.

STEP 2

Turn to chapter 3, "Emotions and Sleep." This chapter reveals how moods and emotional states may interfere with rest and sleep.

Survey the suggestions under the heading "Coping with Emotional States." Pick one that seems to be of particular value, and put it to work. After a week of application, go to Step 3.

STEP 3

Turn to chapter 4, "The Meaning of Dreams." This chapter explores the psychology of the dream process and its relation to REM sleep. The importance of obtaining a sufficient amount of REM sleep is stressed.

Survey the suggestions under the heading "What You Can Do." Pick one that seems to be of particular value, and put it to work. After a week of application, go to Step 4.

STEP 4

Turn to chapter 5, "When Life Is Disorganized." This chapter discusses *sleep hygiene*, the formation of good sleep habits. The assertion is made that positive habits promote system and order; and this in turn promotes relaxation and sleep.

Survey the suggestions under the heading "Acquiring Sleep-Inducing Habits." Pick one that seems to be of particular value, and put it to work. After a week of application, go to Step 5.

STEP 5

Turn to chapter 6, "Self-Hypnosis." This chapter explains what hypnosis is and the nature of self-hypnosis. The point of view is taken that self-hypnosis is a practical sleep-induction skill.

Find the section headed "Using Self-Hypnosis." Under this section you will find a subsection titled "Trance Induction." This provides a step-by-step procedure for learning how to induce a self-hypnotic trance. After a week of application, go to Step 6.

STEP 6

Turn to chapter 7, "More Ways to Obtain Better Sleep." This chapter provides a "catalog" of tips and techniques. For convenient reference, the suggestions have been arranged in alphabetical order.

Select a tip or technique that you believe may be of particular use to you. After a week of application, go to Step 7.

STEP 7

It's time to take a break. For about a week just let go of any conscious or voluntary effort to apply the book's strategies. Take a time out.

About six weeks have passed since you started the program. I hope that the suggestions most applicable to your own difficulties are becoming habits. If you don't feel you need more help to sleep soundly at the present time, place the book on a convenient shelf. Pick up the book when you feel a need to refer to it.

Or, after a week's break, you may want to repeat the seven-step anti-insomnia program. If so, go back to Step 1. This time you might select alternative strategies, making fresh inroads into the problem of insomnia.

The Last Word

The ability to sleep soundly when a person needs to is perceived by human beings in all walks of life as a blessing. When we can't sleep we feel like victims.

If you have a sleep disorder, or suffer from behavioral insomnia, don't despair. You don't have to be a victim if you choose not to. If you assume that you are helpless, that you are doomed to suffer, and that there is no help available, then these very ideas form the basis for a self-defeating, self-fulfilling prophecy.

On the other hand, if you take a positive attitude, if you apply your will and intelligence to the problem of insomnia, you can expect good results. You will find that it is really possible to obtain what *Get a Good Night's Sleep* promises.

Key Points to Remember

- This chapter presented two alternative approaches designed to help you overcome insomnia.

- The first alternative is the *weakest link approach*. Using this approach, you attack sleep difficulties by selecting a group of six or seven suggestions that you believe you can put into immediate and effective action.

- The second alternative is systematic. It is the *seven-step anti-insomnia program* outlined in this chapter.